Religion and
Artificial Reproduction

RELIGION and ARTIFICIAL REPRODUCTION

An Inquiry into the Vatican
"Instruction on Respect for
Human Life in Its Origin and on
the Dignity of Human Reproduction"

THOMAS A. SHANNON
and LISA SOWLE CAHILL

CROSSROAD • NEW YORK

1988
The Crossroad Publishing Company
370 Lexington Avenue, New York, N.Y. 10017

Library of Congress Cataloging-in-Publication Data

Shannon, Thomas A. (Thomas Anthony), 1940–
    Religion and artificial reproduction : an inquiry into the Vatican "Instruction on respect for human life in its origin and on the dignity of human reproduction" / Thomas A. Shannon and Lisa Sowle Cahill.
    p. cm.
    Bibliography: p.
    ISBN 0-8245-0860-2
    1. Catholic Church. Pope (1978– : John Paul II). Instruction on respect for human life in its origin and on the dignity of human reproduction. 2. Human reproduction—Technological innovations—Moral and ethical aspects. 3. Catholic Church—Doctrines.
I. Cahill, Lisa Sowle. II. Title.
QP251.S485 1988
241'.66—dc19
                                                                                    87-30576
                                                                                    CIP

The "Instruction on Respect for Human Life in Its Origin and on the Dignity of Procreation" is reprinted from *Origins* 16, no. 40 (19 March 1987).

To
John R. Connery, S.J.
Richard A. McCormick, S.J.
and
Charles E. Curran

In recognition of their many contributions to
and leadership in Roman Catholic moral theology.

We have not only learned from their writings
but also from their sterling example
of personal integrity and fidelity.

Contents

Preface

We present this book as an introduction to the topic of artificial reproduction, as a commentary on the Vatican document issued in March 1987, "Instruction on Respect for Human Life in Its Origin and on the Dignity of Procreation," and as a discussion of the many complex ethical, social, and political issues that these technologies raise.

Each of the coauthors brings a particular expertise to this topic that he or she has developed through research in both ethical theory and bioethics. To facilitate the writing, the authors took primary responsibility for specific chapters. Thus Lisa Sowle Cahill is the primary author of chapters 2, 5, and 6. Thomas A. Shannon is the primary author of chapters 1, 3, and 4. We have edited each other's chapters and concur with their method and content.

The issues raised by artificial reproduction are complex and difficult and have the potential for transforming the most basic of human relationships. Thus there is a genuine need for a careful examination of these technologies. We hope this contribution will help carry that discussion forward, particularly in the Roman Catholic community, but also for all interested citizens.

1.

A Review of
Artificial Reproduction

Artificial reproduction is not a recent phenomenon, but its application to humans is relatively new. This chapter will review the development and applications of artificial reproduction to provide a context in which our ethical, social, and policy analysis will take place.

In the 1950's, the widespread use of oral contraceptives provided the basis for a sexual revolution. "The Pill," as it came to be known, guaranteed a separation of sexuality from reproduction. By effectively suppressing ovulation, oral contraceptives permitted individuals to have intercourse with an exceptionally high expectation that no pregnancy would occur. And while not all of the sexual excesses of the 1950's and 1960's can be blamed on "The Pill," nonetheless the successful separation of sexual activity from reproduction certainly was a necessary condition for the radical changes of behavior in those decades.

Our generation is experiencing a second sexual revolution that is even more profound and will have as many—if not even more—significant implications for social behavior. Now not only is it possible to have intercourse without reproducing, it is also possible to reproduce without having inter-course.

The first stage of this revolution is rather traditional, es-pecially in animal husbandry, and not too technically com-plex. This is artificial insemination in which sperm is inserted into the female through a syringe or some other device. Its applications to humans have become more common in the last decades, but personal, social, and religious ambiguity still curtails its widespread utilization.

The second stage of the revolution is the technology of *in vitro* fertilization. In this process, an egg and sperm are fer-tilized outside of the female, the fertilized egg cultured and then reimplanted in the uterus. This procedure allows indi-viduals who, for example, are capable of producing eggs and sperm but who have a structural problem such as blocked Fallopian tubes, which prevents impregnation, to bypass the traditional method of fertilization and to establish the preg-nancy technically. The technology is significant for two rea-sons. First, it assists infertile individuals in resolving the issue of childlessness. Second, in the process of externalizing fer-tilization, the embryo is now available for other procedures, such as genetic engineering.

The third stage of the new revolution of reproduction without sexuality utilizes either of the artificial methods of impregnation but has a female who is not the spouse of the male become pregnant and carry the pregnancy for the couple. Such a surrogate mother is used if, for example, the woman is sterile or has a disease that makes pregnancy dangerous for her.

At first glance, these procedures may not look that revo-lutionary, but their implications are profound. Surrogate motherhood, for example, raises profound questions about the definition of mother, the significance of a third party in the marriage, what roles women do or should have, and the impact of this procedure on the children born of it. *In vitro* fertilization raises significant questions about the use to which embryos are put, especially if they are frozen, the regulation of the procedure, the distribution of resources, and how this fits into the traditional practice of medicine. Artificial reproduction also permits lesbians and homosexuals to reproduce without any heterosexual activity whatsoever. At a metaphysical level, these procedures raise the question of the nature of parenthood, the relation of sexuality to marriage, and indeed of the relation of sexuality and reproduction to our very bodiliness. Is reproduction only a matter of volition or need it be in some way an incarnated volitional act?

Many of these and other problems are already coming to the attention of the public. IVF clinics are being established but are guided by no regulations other than the integrity of the staff. Individuals are discussing franchises for reproductive clinics. Embryos are being frozen but, although most clinics require that the donors of the eggs and sperm make some disposition for the embryo, this practice is not mandatory. Questions are being raised about the permissibility of experimentation on *in vitro* embryos or frozen embryos. Agencies have been established to match surrogates with couples wishing a baby. Legislation is being considered in various states and on the federal level. The courts are also being involved, as in the widely publicized case of Baby M in New Jersey in which the biological father and biological mother, not related to each other by marriage, both claimed the child as theirs.

Problems such as these will simply not go away or disappear. As long as the situation continues as it is—especially with its venture-capitalist dimension—we can expect only more difficult and complex problems. Changes in the way we reproduce will have an impact on how we relate to one another, how we understand marriage, and how and where we locate reproduction. In this volume we analyze many of these issues. To situate the debate, we begin with an overview of recent developments in the area of artificial reproduction.

This will provide the technical background for our social, ethical, and religious discussions.

THE HISTORY OF ARTIFICIAL REPRODUCTION

The study of reproduction was greatly aided by the observation of mammalian sperm in the early 1700's and mammalian ova in the early 1800's. These discoveries permitted scientists to break with the traditional and widely held Aristotelian view that the embryo was the product of male seed that was nurtured in the soil of the female. Attempts at *in vitro* fertilization followed soon, with the first recorded attempts occurring in 1878.

Walter Heape was the first, in 1890, successfully to transfer embryos from one mammal to another. Although he was trying to determine what effects, if any, a foster environment would have on the development of offspring and what effects, if any, a foreign embryo might have on the foster mother, Heape established the

> . . . physiological possibility of recovering a preimplantation stage embryo from a female animal by flushing the oviduct, and then transferring the embryo to a foster mother without hindering the development.[1]

This historic work set the stage for applications in various animals including the rat, sheep, and goat in the 1930's, the mouse and cow in the 1940's, the pig in the 1950's, and the horse in the 1970's.[2]

Attention soon focused on the attempt to culture embryos in the laboratory. Nerve cells were cultured in 1907 by Ross Harrison, but it was not until 1958 that A. McLaren and John

Biggers cultured a mouse egg to the blastocyst stage, in which there are approximately fifty cells, and successfully transfered it to a foster mother where it followed a normal course of development.[3] The work of M. Chang made three additional contributions to this developing field. First, he developed a technique for mounting eggs on a slide so they could be evaluated. Second, Chang, in 1951 simultaneously with C. R. Austin, discovered the process of capacitation—a chemical change in the sperm that allows it to penetrate the ovum. Third, in 1959, Chang reported the first documented *in vitro* fertilization and embryo transfer in rabbits through the use of genetic markers.[4]

In 1969 Robert Edwards began his work on the *in vitro* fertilization of human oocytes or eggs. Several technical problems needed to be resolved before Edwards' early low success rates could be increased. Patrick Steptoe's use of laparoscopy, the introduction of a needle under anesthesia through the abdominal wall into the ovary, helped resolve the problem of obtaining ova.[5] The women were injected with "gonadotrophin with follice stimulating hormone (FSH) activity during the early part of the menstrual cycle."[6] This hormone caused superovulation and allowed the recovery of several mature ova as opposed to the one that would typically be mature. Finally, a medium in which the fertilization and maturation could occur was developed. The combination of all these elements, in addition to the investment of much time, energy, and resources, led to the first documented case of an intrauterine human pregnancy following IVF and ET by Edwards and Steptoe on 25 July 1978.

Their efforts were replicated in Australia in 1979, in 1981 in the United States, and quickly thereafter in France, West Germany, England, India, Austria, and South Africa. Thousands of babies have been born through the technique and the method appears to be established.

THE TECHNOLOGIES

What Are They?

A number of methods or technologies are used in artificial reproduction. This section will identify and define them.

Probably the oldest and most simple of the methods of artificial reproduction is artificial insemination. Sperm is obtained typically through masturbation and is either used immediately or is frozen for later use. The sperm are inserted into the cervix whence they move to the Fallopian tubes where fertilization may occur.

Various methods of retrieving ova have been developed. Typically several ova are induced into maturing through the use of hormones. They are then obtained through laparoscopy. After sperm and egg are obtained, they are combined in a medium and, after the capacitation of the sperm occurs, fertilization can occur. This is *in vitro* fertilization (IVF). After reaching an appropriate level of maturity, the preembryo is then transferred through the cervix to the prepared uterus of the woman in the expectation that it will implant and develop. This process is called embryo transfer (ET). Since several ova are fertilized simultaneously but not used, many individuals began freezing the embryos so they would not be destroyed and to have them available for future attempts to establish pregnancies. This is called cryopreservation or cryostorage.[7]

There are some variations on these techniques. For example, one team establishes a pregnancy through artificial insemination and then loosens the embryo through lavage (washing the uterus with a solution), collects it in a specially designed catheter and then reinserts the embryo into the prepared uterus of a woman who has tubal infertility but a functioning uterus. The procedure of gamete intra-Fallopian transfer (GIFT) is used in women who have normal Fallopian tubes but are infertile because of, for example, unexplained infertility or an immunologic response to the male. The ovaries are hyperstimulated and ova retrieved as in IVF. Then the ova and sperm are placed in a catheter in proximity to each other and are reinserted into the Fallopian tube so insemination can occur *in vivo.*[8] A similar method is low tubal ovum transfer (LTOT), which is designed for women with blocked Fallopian tubes. Here the same initial procedures as in IVF are followed to retrieve the ova, but they are reimplanted lower in the Fallopian tube so the blockage will not interfere with the possibility of conception *in vivo.*[9]

Unspecified by the technologies is the source of the gametes and to whom the preembryo is returned. The technologies enable or facilitate fertilization. Social-ethical questions emerge from various applications of the technologies, for example surrogate motherhood in which a woman may be artificially inseminated by a male who is not her spouse. She then carries the pregnancy and relinquishes the child to the male and his spouse for them to raise. Alternatively, ova or a frozen preembryo can be donated to an infertile couple. Thus the technologies make possible a variety of combinations of pregnancy and parenthood.

Risks

TO THE EMBRYO?

One of the first concerns with artificial reproduction was that the techniques used could present a risk of harm to the embryo. Several studies have addressed this problem, and the overall conclusion is that the techniques do not present an increased risk of harm. This is not to say that children born of the methods of artificial reproduction may not have some problems but that the likelihood of their being caused by the process of conception is minimal.

John D. Biggers first reported on risk factors in a 1981 article.[10] Because few children had as yet been born of IVF and ET, few data were available. Biggers identified four ways in which abnormalities could be increased:

> the induction of chromosomal aberrations, an increase in the rate of fertilization by abnormal spermatozoa, the induction of point mutations, and the actions of physical and chemical teratogens.[11]

This essentially means that harm to the fertilized egg can be caused by a chemical used in the procedure, having fertilization occur through sperm that are not normal, introducing a change in the structure of the organism at a particular point, and through the use of some chemical in the solution or through, for example, the method by which the organism is reinserted in the uterus. He noted that animal studies indicated increased incidences of risks in these areas, but the transfer to humans is unclear. Thus, while Biggers recognized that the technologies may cause an increase of defects, he said the evidence "suggests that the danger of increased congenital defects is not high."[12]

Biggers reviewed the data again in 1983, this time with a sample of over 125 children born of IVF and ET.[13] This study indicated that the procedures presented little risk to the embryo. Biggers indicated that in general there is at birth about a 1 percent risk of congenital defects, which increases by a factor of about three in the first five years.[14] Of the first 125 births from IVF and ET, Biggers said that "only one case of a congenital defect has occurred."[15] Since other defects may manifest themselves only later, however, follow-up studies must be done. Another study also concludes that "there is no evidence that simple mutations [changes in the gene structure] and teratogenic effects [harm to the structure caused by some agent or procedure] can be attributed to IVF techniques."[16]

John Yovich and others undertook a developmental assessment of IVF infants at their first birthday, including a general pediatric history and a review of any significant events.[17] Previously the infants were studied at birth by two pediatricians and assessed during the neonatal period. Of the twenty infants, three had fetal abnormalities. The problems of one infant were resolved spontaneously and another's were corrected surgically. The third had a deformed right external ear, two extra ribs, and Goldenhar's syndrome.[18] Based on their scoring system, only one infant in the twenty had a corrected assessment score of below 100, with the overall corrected average being 117.48.[19]

Given these studies, one can reasonably conclude that IVF and ET present only a minimal, if indeed any at all, risk of harm to the embryo. As the data base grows larger, however, monitoring should continue to determine whether these early results will be verified over time.

TO THE WOMAN?

The birth technologies present a variety of risks to the woman in addition to the more general risks associated with the infertility work-up itself. These general risks include the adverse effects of the loss of the privacy and intimacy of one's sexual life during the time of infertility testing. An endometrial biopsy, which requires a scraping of the uterus with a sharp instrument to obtain tissues for examination, is often required. The uterus and oviducts may also be filled with a dye and then x-rayed to find irregularities in these structures. In addition, there may be hormonal treatments to help various systems function correctly. These procedures are often painful, the infections occasionally associated with them may decrease fertility, and the woman may need to undergo them frequently.

With respect to IVF, the first risk is biochemical and is caused by the use of hormones to induce superovulation to enhance the possibility of obtaining several ova. There appear to be no short-term risks associated with this, but studies should be done to monitor any potential long-term effects. Edwards notes that such stimulation which results in high levels

> of plasma progesterone in the luteal phase, may lead to disorders in uterine development, and this point has not been satisfactorily established in any clinic as far as I am aware.[20]

A second set of risks derives from the method of retrieval of the oocytes. Frequently a laparoscopy is required, during which time the woman must be under general anesthesia and is subject to the risks of that which are quite low. Occasionally a prior laparoscopy is required because the ovary, caught in adhesions, is inaccessible.[21] More recently, however, ultrasound aspiration is being utilized to obtain ova, and this will reduce the need for general anesthesia.[22]

A third set of risks are physical. The major risk is the 2 to 4 percent chance of an ectoptic pregnancy occurring after ET, a percentage ". . . much higher than found in the normal fertile population."[23] While such a risk may not be higher than that for other infertile populations, such pregnancies present a life-threatening situation for the mother, in addition to a threat to the life of the embryo. The cervix may also be obstructed during the attempt to insert the catheter, which reduces the chance of establishing a pregnancy. Such difficulties may also cause bleeding with associated pain, which can cause anxiety. This may lower the woman's pain threshold, thereby increasing the pain.[24] Also, pregnancy may be monitored more intensively and, while ultrasound has no known risk factor and amniocentesis carries a small risk of miscarriage, both may provoke anxiety and discomfort. Finally, many of the pregnancies are delivered by Caesarean section. In one study, six of the infants, or 50 percent of the study, were delivered in this fashion.[25] Whether this method of delivery is used primarily to ensure a safe delivery for a pregnancy in which so much has been invested or because it is medically appropriate is unclear.

Finally, there are psychological risks. The procedures associated with infertility work-ups are anxiety-producing and can cause strain on the spouses' relationship.[26] Also the couple is frequently disappointed because the procedure does not resolve their childlessness.[27]

Thus the procedures associated with IVF and ET carry some degree of risk—mainly of morbidity—with them. The major life-threatening risk is that of the ectopic pregnancy. The others fall within the normal risks associated with medical examinations and minor procedures.

Benefits

The benefits of the birth technologies are clear and direct: the individuals have a child that is related to one or both of them, depending on the origin of the gametes. The reproductive technologies resolve the problem of childlessness by providing a means for an infertile couple to have a child. Thus, even though one or both of the individuals remain infertile, they have the experience of pregnancy and have a child related genetically to at least one of them.

Another benefit is diagnostic. The couple may learn the cause of the infertility and, on that basis, eliminate various options before they are emotionally committed to them. Thus if infertility is a consequence of male-factor infertility, IVF with the husband's sperm is unlikely to be successful.

As such, the technologies resolve the frustrations and anxieties that childlessness brings. A major source of stress is removed from the couple and strains on their lives and relationship are ended. The resolution and relief of all sorts of psychological as well as physical problems and sources of anxiety must be counted among the benefits of the reproductive technologies.

Success Rate

Since the obtaining of a child is the primary benefit of IVF, one needs to know how often this event will occur. That is, what is the success rate of the various technologies?

To answer this, several factors will have to be examined. First, what counts as pregnancy? A distinction is made between a chemical or biochemical pregnancy and a clinical pregnancy. A biochemical pregnancy occurs when ". . . there is a significant rise in the β-HCG [human chorionic gonadotropin] level."[28] This test reports the presence of a pregnancy by evaluating the presence and level of hormones associated with the establishment of a pregnancy. A clinical pregnancy is one in which there is ". . . both endocrinologic and clinical evidence of pregnancy."[29] Establishing what a particular clinic or physician uses as a criterion of pregnancy is thus an important first step in determining the success of the program.

One of the most difficult problems is the determination of the rate of success. There is no one standard that all use in reporting the results of IVF. Thus some report success per chemical pregnancy, success per laparoscopy, success per implantation, etc. Infrequently reported, however, is the actual number of live births. What will be presented here, then, is a representative sample of success rates and the basis on which these are calculated.

The first comprehensive study of the success of IVF was done by Clifford Grobstein in 1983. At that time, the clinical field was young and the data were easier to gather. For example, Grobstein reported on thirteen centers.[30] In 1986, the Registry in the *Journal of In Vitro Fertilization and Embryo Transfer* listed 140 centers. Thus increased volume as well as the absence of a single accepted criterion of success make record-keeping difficult.

Grobstein used three measures of success: the number of pregnancies, the pregnancies per laparoscopy, and pregnancies per embryo transfer. Grobstein reported a total of 2,037 laparoscopies and 1,110 embryo transfers. On a pregnancy per laparoscopy basis, there were 166 pregnancies. On a pregnancy per embryo-transfer basis, there were 310 pregnancies. This gives an efficacy of 8 percent for pregnancies per laparoscopy and 16.5 percent for pregnancies per embryo transfer.[31] Grobstein concludes that the success rate of ET is about 40 percent that of traditional fertilization.[32] Absent is the actual number of children born.

The experiences of many clinics are now being reported and these show a wide range of successes and failures. The Monash–Queen Victoria Medical Centre published their rates from July-December 1981.[33] Of 126 total laparoscopies, there were 101 embryo transfers and nineteen pregnancies. The pregnancy per total laparoscopy rate was 15 percent and the pregnancy per embryo-transfer rate was 19 percent.

Success rates are also calculated by pregnancy per number of laparoscopies. Sixty-eight patients had one laparoscopy each resulting in seven pregnancies; the success rate is 10 percent. Thirty-five patients had two laparoscopies each resulting in seven pregnancies for a success rate of 20 percent; fourteen patients had three laparoscopies, resulting in four pregnancies for a success rate of 29 percent. Two had four laparoscopies resulting in one pregnancy with a success rate of 50 percent. Finally, one patient had five laparoscopies but did not become pregnant.

The success rates are also reported on a pregnancy per embryo-transfer basis. Here seventy-nine patients received one embryo each, resulting in sixteen pregnancies for a 16 percent success rate. Nineteen received two embryos each which resulted in three pregnancies for a rate of 16 percent. Finally, five patients received three embryos each and the success rate went to 60 percent.[34] This last datum represents a widespread clinical observation: the more embryos one implants—up to around four or five—the higher the success rate.

Another study at Monash reported on an eighteen-month study of 204 patients who had a total of 204 embryo transfers. This study was primarily interested in the type of catheter used in the ET; so the number of laparoscopies was not reported. Thirty-four pregnancies resulted. A further 127 patients, not included in this study but using techniques derived from the study, had 152 transfers, resulting in seventeen clinical pregnancies.[35]

Patrick Steptoe reported on statistics from 1 January 1981 to 20 March 1982 in his practice at Bourne Hall. During this time, 726 patients underwent 751 laparoscopies; of these, 625 had ova recovered.[36] A total of 527 fertilizations *in vitro* were established and 507 embryo transfers occurred. From these, 101 pregnancies occurred (86 biochemical and 15 biochemical) from which came sixty-two children from sixty births. According to Steptoe, the 101 pregnancies represent 20 percent of the embryo transfers and 14 percent of the patients.[37] Thus, from 751 laparoscopies in 726 patients, there were sixty-two live births.

The program at Eastern Virginia Medical School (EVMS) has been in place since 1981. During that time, the success rate for pregnancy has risen from 12.7 percent in 1981 to 26.7 percent in 1985. In addition, the success rate based on cycles of transfer has increased from 21.4 percent in 1981 to 28.1 percent in 1985. Finally, the pregnancy rate also varies with the number of ova implanted: 21 percent in the transfer of a single fertilized egg, to 30 percent with two, and 40+ percent with three mature eggs.[38] Professor Gary Hodgen of EVMS recently reported that ". . . for each treatment cycle about 230 babies will be delivered."[39] Additionally at EVMS

". . . the cummulative pregnancy rate after three (3) IVF treatment cycles exceeds 50 percent."[40]

Another study reports on success rates at six of Australia's IVF centers.[41] By the middle of 1982, 131 pregnancies were reported from 1,581 embryo transfers. The ova came from 4,554 follicle aspirations during 1,660 laparoscopies, with an average of 2.3 ova obtained per laparoscopy. These pregnancies resulted in forty live births, with three mothers delivering twins.

Finally, a recent article in *The New York Times* indicates that since 1981, eight hundred babies have been born in the United States through IVF and that in 1986, about six thousand IVF fertilizations took place.[42] In addition about 150 clinics have been established, with about sixty-five of them at university centers. Of these clinics, a physician claimed that only a handful—"perhaps as few as six"[43] are responsible for about two-thirds of the total births.

What is clear from this review of several studies is that the success rates of pregnancy either per laparoscopy or per embryo transfer are increasing. It is clear that transfering multiple fertilized ova also increases the success rate. Yet there is still a large gap between fertilization, embryo transfer, and live births. For example, using the live birth per laparoscopy measure, the success rate of Steptoe is 8.2 percent. And in the Australian study of six hospitals, the success rate of live birth per laparoscopy is 2.4 percent, and the success rate per embryo transfer is 2.5 percent. Thus, while some success rates increase, the critical statistic is still the number of children actually born, and that number appears to be quite low. However, many of the losses are miscarriages, some a consequence of an ectopic pregnancy and some a second- or third-trimester pregnancy loss, as can occur in a pregnancy established customarily. What is clear is that success needs to be defined more clearly and statistics need to be maintained so that a better overall picture can be obtained.

Cost of the Procedure

Another datum that is difficult to obtain is the actual cost of the procedure. The difficulty is determining what to include as a cost. For example, should lost wages, meals, and lodging be included?

The 1983 study by Grobstein included a section on costs based on estimates from the EVMS. At that time, the cost for the screening to enter the program was $2,465 and the cost for the actual procedure was $5,590.[44] Thus the initial attempt costs a little over $8,000. Each additional attempt costs another $5,000. Assuming an overall efficiency rate of 10 percent,

> . . . something of the order of $38,000 would be required to ensure a roughly 50 percent chance of a live birth for a particular patient. For each child born, aggregate costs are about $50,000, borne by both the successful and unsuccessful couples.[45]

Another set of sample costs is available for an Australian program current for 1982. Here the cost for one treatment cycle of IVF and ET is $1,512.60 (Australian).[46] These costs are medical in that they include only the costs of the materials, the personnel, the surgical theater, and a three-day admission to the hospital. When travel, lodging, and lost wages are included, the costs would increase, but probably not to the level of the American costs.[47]

A critical factor in costs, obviously, is whether insurance, either private or public, is available for the procedure. For example, Traveler's, Aetna, and Blue Shield have "premium waivers that cover up to four treatments . . ."[48] Kaiser Permanente also supports some IVF costs. How these insurance issues will be resolved by other carriers is yet to be determined and will be part of the next major debate surrounding artificial reproduction.

IVF is a growth industry with an estimated "$30 to $40 million market in IVF procedures . . ."[49] In addition, sales of ultrasound equipment with special probes for a noninvasive retrieval of ova are expected to rise from the present $5 million to $35 million within a few years. Start-up costs of a clinic are high, however, with about $1 million being necessary to produce an efficiently run program.[50] This requires a high patient volume which in turn necessitates marketing to bring in the patients. Some clinics have offered public stock to raise revenue. "In Vitro Care, Inc., organized by doctors in Cambridge, Mass., for example, raised over $4 million is a public stock offering on October 1985, but has yet to open a clinic."[51] Others are attempting to gain a monopoly on a special procedure involving embryo donation. In this procedure a woman is artifically inseminated and the embryo given to another woman who then carries the pregnancy and raises the child. Fertility and Genetics Research, Inc. of Chicago ". . . has been awarded a patent on instruments to retrieve eggs and has applied for a patent on the entire medical procedure."[52]

Thus, in addition to the competition to develop the best procedures and obtain the best success rates, there is also a great deal of competition to secure patients and money. When one combines these unregulated activities with the desperation of individuals to have children, there is a high potential for the exploitation of infertile couples.

Impact on the Patients

The fact of involuntary infertility is a well-documented cause of stress and anxiety in couples and individuals.[53] Participation in a program that offers the resolution of childlessness can only increase the stress and anxiety already felt, especially if the couple appreciates fully the low success rates.

Entering an IVF program is not usually the couple's first

attempt to resolve infertility or childlessness. They typically have been through series of tests, studies, and procedures. This group is ". . . vulnerable, desperate, anxious, and under both physiological and psychological stress."[54] In addition, the experience of undergoing IVF may involve the couple in ". . . far more stress in a relatively short period of time than the couple has experienced before."[55] Thus the couple are in a rather vulnerable situation, to which attention must be given.

Studies differ, however, on the emotional state of individuals and couples entering a program. A Canadian study, for example, reports that on the Family Environment Scale, IVF couples ". . . indicated significantly greater organization, cohesion, expressiveness, and a stronger moral-religious emphasis in their relationship."[56] On the Quality of Life Questionnaire, they ". . . reported higher levels of personal growth, marital relation, extended family relations, extrafamilial relation, job characteristics, job satisfiers, and vacation behavior than the normative group."[57] Thus, the study concludes, ". . . the majority of couples entering an *in vitro* fertilization program will present with normal personality functioning."[58] On the other hand, another study reports that individuals

> . . . conceal anxiety and emotional distress in initial assessments (consciously and/or unconsciously) because of fears that candor will result in their exclusion from the program.[59]

Clearly one needs to identify one's population so that one can respond to their needs. For example, if the majority have normally functioning personalities, but have ". . . high needs for orderly, predictable, threat-free environments that offer them opportunity for support,"[60] then one needs to ensure a continuous flow of information and mechanisms of support.

On the other hand, since there are some inherent elements of stress— ". . . the waiting list, the cost, the low success rates, the end-of-the-line implication of IVF and the medical demands of the program"[61]—discussions of them up front may prepare individuals to deal with the stress that is certain to come.

Several other causes of stress have also been identified. One is the uncertainty that comes from not knowing whether the procedure was successful or not.[62] In addition, the experience can be emotionally draining.[63] The procedure also generates anxiety.[64] This is because of the hope the procedure offers and because it may be a couple's last chance to resolve their childlessness. Stress also comes from unrealistic expectations for success, even though the individuals have been informed of the success rates.[65] Thus, because IVF is the last hope, it must be successful and even the possibility of its failure is difficult to accept.

Two other factors are critical. First, a grief reaction may follow the failure of IVF.[66] This reaction can include bodily distress, guilt feelings, and hostility to others. The reaction is similar to the experience of miscarriage and apparently occurs because some ". . . view embryo transfer as a pregnancy."[67] A grief reaction based on this perception can last for several weeks and can cause prolonged periods of crying, loss of appetite, and poor sleep. Second, for a subset of patients for whom IVF was unsuccessful, other alternatives to biological parenthood are unacceptable. In one study 93 percent said they would participate in ". . . any innovative methods for achieving a biological pregnancy."[68] This suggests a strong urge to have a biological child and a ". . . readiness to jump on the bandwagon of new reproductive programs."[69] These factors would confer a particular obligation on the staff of such programs to ensure that individuals are adequately informed of the success rates, risks, etc., for any new programs that are offered. This population appears to be quite vulnerable and perhaps even desperate. Thus they may need to be protected against themselves.

A final issue is the stress level of the staff. The patients, even though they know the success rates are low, assume they will become pregnant. This puts pressure on the staff and also causes them to identify with the couples' feelings of failure in achieving a pregnancy. Staff members themselves can become frustrated with the low success rates. Thus the small number of successes may not be enough to give ". . . the continuous positive reenforcement of the staff that is necessary for their morale."[70] Especially in small programs, the staff's needs, as well as the patients', must be attended to in order to ensure the atmosphere necessary for the harmonious running of the program.

CONCLUSIONS

IVF is a rapidly growing field. Programs are expanding quickly and numerious individuals are utilizing the procedure. IVF has proven to be a safe technology, presenting few risks to the woman and minimal risks to the conceptus. Yet, success rates are low, even in the best programs. The success rates of the best programs are between 25 to 30 percent, but some programs have yet to achieve a pregnancy. From the perspective of the number of live births, the success rates are even lower.

As the practice continues, experience grows, and research is more focused, more successes will be attained and more will be learned. But such knowledge and success may also succeed in adding new layers of complications and quandaries to the ethical dilemmas we already face. How we shall deal with these remains to be seen. But clearly, the technologies are here to stay.[71]

2.

Sexuality, Marriage, and Parenthood: The Catholic Tradition

New methods of controlling the reproductive process by means of technical intervention pose challenges to ethical interpretation, not only of human sexuality and conception, but also of what it means to be a parent and a spouse. The Christian tradition offers resources for assessment of new reproductive possibilities, because those possibilities arise from and revise fundamental human relationships that have always been matters of key importance for Christian moral reflection. There already exists a well-refined tradition concerning the human and Christian meanings of sexual activity; marriage as a sexual, domestic, and social partnership; and the activity of procreation, which joins the spousal relationship to the parental one, creating the family. This tradition has varied over time, is not always consistent, and has received challenges as well as reaffirmations in the twentieth century. If the usefulness of this tradition is to continue, its key elements must be clarified, then reexamined and reinterpreted in the light of the particular historical and cultural context to which the tradition is to speak.

What lies at the heart of a Christian, and especially a Catholic, teaching on sexuality, marriage, and parenthood? Elements that many would readily identify as "Roman Catholic" teaching could include the following: Marriage is a sacrament, one consequence of which is that it is "indissoluble." This is the basis of the prohibition of divorce and remarriage within Catholicism. Historically, marriage has taken second place to virginity or celibacy, typically lived out in religious congregations or orders. The marriage of Mary and Joseph, traditionally held to be celibate, was proposed as the ideal. A celibate lifestyle was said to free one totally to serve God. In addition, there is the lingering suspicion or belief that sexual intercourse represents a sort of capitulation to physical drives or passions.

A spiritual life can be accomplished through marriage, however. Above all, what makes this possible is fidelity to one's spouse, the birth of children, their education, and the handing on of the faith to them. In this context, procreation is the primary purpose of sex. Any attempt artificially to prevent procreation is wrong. The only allowable method of birth control is rhythm, which makes use of the natural infertile period. Finally, all sexual activity other than heterosexual relations open to procreation within the context of sacramental marriage is prohibited. All other sexual acts are evaluated according to the same standard; all are objectively and mortally sinful.

In this overview, "marriage" consistently appears as the inclusive category, overarching and containing the meanings of sexuality and parenthood. Marriage is the only appropriate context for either (excepting some of the parental relations created by adoption), and it is parenthood that really justifies sex, even within marriage. The existence of sexual activity outside this context is addressed mainly in terms of restrictive prohibitions. Yet sex can be good and even holy if placed in its proper setting. Many also are aware that the Church recently has condemned reproductive technologies, but do not understand fully why this follows from the stated premises (especially given the centrality of procreation). They perhaps also would not realize that technologies even within marriage, as well as those involving donors or "surrogates," are rejected.

Most Catholics, as well as non-Catholic onlookers, are aware that "Catholic" teaching emanates from some unitary, official source, especially "the Pope." Many Catholics assume as well that papal teaching is grounded on and repeats what the Bible says. Personal disagreement with some of these teachings—in theory or in practice—can lead to a serious crisis of faith, to overwhelming guilt over unresolved conflict between the perceived requirements of religious obedience and those of personal moral experience, or—as in the case of many younger Catholics—to alienation from the Church. Non-Catholics, who often appeal to the Bible in support of rather different views, take issue with some of the above propositions, seeing them as rooted in irrational religious authoritarianism and as fundamentally damaging to human happiness and harmony in the realms of sexuality and of marriage. In particular, contemporary criticisms are aimed at indissolubility, the Church's unwavering rejections of artificial contraception and of sex outside heterosexual marriage, and the limitation of means of procreation to "natural" sexual acts between spouses.

This hypothetical "popular" view of these matters is not entirely accurate; neither is it entirely misguided. Certainly there is in the Christian tradition an ingrained suspicion about the goodness of sexuality and a fear of its tendency to escape orderly expression and become destructive. This negative perspective combines with the positive insight that marriage contributes to the order and prosperity of human society, and with it creates a focus on procreation as a good outcome of sexual acts, a good which contributes to the welfare of the parents, the family, and of society as a whole. It is true that many traditional authors, such as Augustine and Aquinas, saw procreation as the foremost justification of sex, but they did not see it as the only purpose of marriage. The union of spouses as such makes its own social and domestic contribution, and serves to direct and order sexual needs. The Catholic Church since the Second Vatican Council no longer gives a "primary" place to procreation in speaking of the "purposes" of sex, nor does it hedge in sexual experience with so much negative language.

The major modern shift in the Catholic understanding of sex is to link it in an equally fundamental way with the interpersonal communion (love) of the partners, and so to give it an intrinsically positive meaning. Prohibitions of divorce, contraception, reproduction technologies, and extramarital sex are not ends in themselves. They are grounded affirmatively—or are at least claimed to be—in the unitive and mutual "self-giving" of the partners through a physical act with a symbolic interpersonal meaning and a natural potential for the creation of new persons.

Another often-unrecognized characteristic of the Catholic teaching about sexuality, parenthood, and marriage is that it is not lodged fundamentally in religious authority, either biblical or papal. Its primary source is an understanding of *natural human values,* developed over centuries in close contact both with certain key scriptural passages and with past traditions and theological interpretations of the Church. Sometimes these confluent streams are difficult to strain apart. But their common theme in addressing moral values is an appreciation of creation, and of created human nature as good, despite the inevitability of sin. Humans retain the ability to reflect on their experience, recognize what is morally required of them, and then to find confirmation of natural moral values in the teachings of and traditions about Jesus. A major cause of confusion about exactly what it is that defines a "Catholic Christian" perspective on any moral issue—including issues of sexual morality—is unclarity on many sides about the precise relation that does or should exist among concrete experiences, reasonable generalizations about the meaning and value of human experience, apparently relevant scriptural insights, and Church teaching on an issue. Church teaching—especially that which originates in the Vatican—usually presents itself as giving adequate and appropriate recognition to concrete experience, reasonable ethical reflection, scripture, and Christian tradition, and as deriving its conclusions from these resources in combination. On some issues, even some persons whose basic loyalties are with the Church find the presentation unconvincing. A firm authoritative stance combined with an unpersuaded audience can lead to doubt and divisiveness. No clear and obvious solution to impasses of this sort seems at hand, even in an area so important as sexual morality. This chapter proceeds on the assumption that nuance enhances knowledge, knowledge enhances understanding, and that understanding facilitates consensus or at least cooperation. We aim here to elucidate the continuity of and variation within Catholic Christian approaches to sexuality, marriage, and parenthood, and thus to contribute to dialogue, both with the tradition and with proponents of the new reproduction technologies.

BIBLICAL RESOURCES

Although the basic foundation of Catholic ethics as "natural-law" ethics is common human wisdom rather than revelation, the Catholic tradition presupposes that essential human values will not be inconsistent with Christian ones. In addition, biblical narratives, images, and injunctions are appropriate for use within the religious community, in shaping a moral identity and providing motivation for living up to those ideals that should in principle be visible to every reasonable human moral intelligence. Since Catholic ethics is also always a Christian ethics, it looks to the biblical witness in order to clarify the ideals to which humans ought aspire and which are given a particular coloring in the life and teaching of Jesus.

Hebrew Bible

Diversity in the roots of our religious understanding of sexuality and marriage begins at least as early as the Hebrew tradition. Existing somewhat in tension with each other are at least two traditions about sex and two about the proper relation between men and women. Throughout the Hebrew Bible, sex is seen as a positive part of creation. While its purpose generally is understood to be the production of heirs who will continue the tribal and religious community, it is at least occasionally portrayed (for example, in the Song of Songs) as an avenue of the mutual delight of lovers. Corresponding to this duality about sex is a duality about women. The Hebrew tradition is essentially patriarchal, as evidenced by the male genealogies that provide continuity to its history (Gen. 5,12). The "forefathers" are Abraham, Isaac, and Jacob. The story of the Exodus is to be retold to the "sons" of Israel (Ex. 12:24). Women have their identity through males, and especially through their childbearing role (see the story of Abraham, Sarah, and Hagar and their children in Genesis 16 and 21. However, recent feminist studies[1] of the Genesis creation stories (Gen. 1:27–28, and 2:7–25) have demonstrated that the original design of the Creator may have been otherwise. Men and women were created for equal partnership, and sexual hierarchy is the result of sin (Gen. 3:1–24).

In describing the creation of humanity, the book of Genesis portrays a God who is active in history, who is immediately involved in making and caring for the human creature, who delegates responsibility to that creature, and who calls humans to account for disobedience and willful failure. Sexual differentiation is part of what it means to be human; the sexes are to cooperate in procreation, in mutual help and companionship, and in fulfilling the tasks that God assigns to humanity within the world. Genesis 1 contains the more terse account:

> So God created man in his own image, in the image of God he created him; male and female he created them. And God blessed them, and God said to them, "Be fruitful and multiply and fill the earth and subdue it; and have dominion over the fish of the sea and over the birds of the air and over every living thing that moves upon the earth." (vv. 26–28)

Within this text, both male and female are associated with "man" or humanity, and thus with creation in the image of God. Further, to both are addressed the "blessing of increase" and the privilege and responsibility of "dominion."

The second (but chronologically earlier) creation story takes a more extended narrative form and tells of the individual creation of the man and the woman, or of an initial human creature, and a later differentiation into two sexes by the addition of a creature of the same human nature but different sex. God formed "man" (human being) "of dust from the ground, and breathed into his nostrils the breath of life" (Gen. 2:7). Recognizing that it is "not good that the man should be alone," God resolves "to make him a helper fit for him" (v. 18). After trying out the different varieties of beast, God finally realizes that they will not serve his purpose. As with the first creature, God works with a raw material that he molds into a new creation. As he produced the first from dust, he now makes the woman from a rib of the man (vv. 21–22). Finally satisfied, the man exclaims, "This at last is bone of my bones and flesh of my flesh" (v. 23). The narrator adds that for this reason men and women leave their families of origin to form a new partnership, in which each "cleaves" to the other and "become one flesh" (v. 24). The second account does not mention procreation but contributes instead the importance of human existence in two sexes for social and domestic partnership and for companionship. The narrative militates against any idea that sex is not in itself good, or that its sole purpose is continuation of the species. Taken together, the creation accounts emphasize the equality and mutual, committed cooperation of men and women as the precondition of their fulfillment of God's commands.

The debacle of Genesis 3 is unhappily familiar. Discontent with faithful obedience to the source of their life and prosperity, the couple listen to the serpent's sophistry and eat of the fruit that the Lord God has forbidden. Less frequently noted is the fact that the woman takes the initiative and discourses with the serpent, while the man abdicates personal responsibility and merely does as she suggests. Both try to evade blame when discovered by God, but eventually are judged guilty and sent from the Garden. Only now does God say to the leader in the sinful eating of fruit that her husband shall "rule over" her, and that she shall suffer "pain in childbearing" (v. 16); and, with equal ironic reversal, to the follower, that he shall henceforth have to exert himself "in toil" and "in the sweat of your face" in order to "eat"—not "of the tree" as previously but "of the ground"—"thorns and thistles," "plants," and "bread" (vv. 17–19). Only after the fact of sin and as its consequence do we find the introduction of sexual hierarchy and the suggestion of gender roles; both are signs and causes of suffering, not part of the design in the good creation.

The egalitarian ideal that Genesis distinguishes from and sets before sin was achieved neither in the patriarchal social organization of ancient Israel nor in the Hebrew scriptures as a whole. Women are distinctly subordinate and their roles are determined by their status in relation to men: as daughters, wives, mothers. The meaning of sexuality takes its coloring from the social relations of those who participate in it. Since women are no longer the equal companions and partners of men, their primary function is to bear children who continue the male line, and this too becomes the major function of sex and of marriage. Laws regulating sexuality and marriage reflect concern with the production of heirs and with certainty of lineage, as well as Israel's patriarchal social structure. Marriage in Israel could be polygamous (polygynous) until about the time of the monarchy in the tenth century B.C. (Gen. 29:21–30, II Sam. 5:13–16, I Kg. 11:1, 3). Marriage could be dissolved by divorce at the initiative of the husband only (Dt. 24:1–4, but see a contrary example in Mal. 2:14–16). Even alongside monogamous marriage, the practices of concubinage (Gen. 16:1–4, 30:1–13) and levirate marriage (Gen. 38:8, Dt. 25:5–10) existed in order to guarantee that men would have heirs, and also that status as childbearers could be ensured even for infertile women and widows. Sex outside of the marriage relation was prohibited, and more stringently so for women, since the legitimacy of a man's children had to be certain. If a man committed adultery with a prostitute his action was not punishable by law, although he was warned against such actions as imprudent and ultimately self-defeating (Pr. 5; 7:5, 25–27). Adultery of a wife or a betrothed virgin was punishable with the death penalty for both partners (Lev. 20:10, Dt. 22:22–27). Despite this male-centered framework for understanding sexuality, marriage, and even parenthood, several prominent women appear in the biblical literature, though they rarely are permitted to overshadow their male counterparts: Rebekah, Sarah, Hagar, Rachel, Leah, Zipporah, Deborah, Naomi, Ruth, Abigail, and Judith. Even in the patriarchal family, the ideal wife demonstrated integrity and enterprise, contributing to the social and economic welfare of the household (Pr. 31:3–31). A counterpoint to the marital and parental meanings of sexuality is offered in the Song of Songs (Song of Solomon). In this erotic poem, replete with luxuriant pastoral imagery, two lovers longingly prepare for and anticipate their union—quite apart from any mention of parenthood or marriage!

In the Hebrew Bible as a whole, then, pregnancy and birth are seen as important, even paramount goods. Children are blessings from God and signs of his favor. Parenthood is especially important for individuals because, in the absence of any definite religious belief in an afterlife, women and especially men looked for immortality through their children and their children's children. Perhaps even more essential to its importance is the contribution procreation makes to the religious community as the covenant people of God. It is heirs who make possible the survival of the Chosen People and the continuation of the covenant God has established with them. It is within the religious rituals of the community that the gracious action of God in the Exodus from slavery in Egypt is commemorated and communal identity reinforced. Women are not the primary participants in this historical mediation of identity, but they have an essential role in it through their capacity to bear children and to make domestic contributions to social and religious survival.

New Testament and Early Christianity

In the Christian biblical literature, quite a different picture emerges. The importance of kinship, marriage, and parenthood diminishes drastically, although their fundamental goodness is certainly not denied. The identity of the religious community is no longer a national or tribal one. The community is not created or even sustained through family inheritance of the faith. Indeed Jesus was a scandal to his fellow Jews because he reached beyond the bounds of Jewish identity to preach the "good news" of God's mercy and of the approaching kingdom. Gentiles too could be included in the coming reign of God if they were obedient to God's will by imitating his forgiveness and doing good to those in need (Mt. 5–7). For Jesus and his first followers, the gospel is spread and the community formed by conversion and not by family membership, and the community of disciples is potentially universal. One's relation to God is no longer tied closely to marital, familial, or racial status (Mk. 3:31–35; Lk. 8:19–21; Mt. 12:46–50; Mk. 10:37; Lk. 14:26). Added to this iconoclastic message is the fact that primitive Christianity expected the eschatological reign of God to be completed in the first generation, which made the question of believers' future children less important and gave emphasis to celibacy.

Nonetheless, marriage and parenthood are not rejected as Christian states of life. The institutions of marriage and family provide a background to many of Jesus' teachings and deeds, and he concurred that adultery constitutes a violation of a legitimate bond (Jn. 8:3–11; Mt. 5:27–28). A prevalent tradition portrays Jesus' repudiation of the contemporary Jewish practice of divorce (Mk. 10:11–12; Mt. 5:31–32, 19:9; Lk. 16:18; 1 Cor. 7:10–11), in which he cites the "one flesh" unity of woman and man established at the creation (Mt. 19:3–8, Mk. 10:2–9), and insists that fidelity obligates both wife and husband. The major theme of Jesus' teaching, however, is not morality, but conversion to the kingdom through repentance and faith (Mk. 1:14–15).

The equality of male and female that is reflected in Jesus' unwillingness to give the husband any special prerogatives vis-à-vis divorce seems also to have been a presupposition of his ministry. At least for a first-century Jew, his actions toward women were radical. He spoke with them, taught them, and included them among his first disciples. Contrary to the typical and unbiblical stereotype, all four gospels portray Mary Magdalene among the first witnesses to the resurrection (Mk. 16:9–11; Lk. 24:1–11; Mt. 28:1–10; Jn. 20:14–18). According to the account in Matthew's, and even more clearly in John's, gospels she also fulfills the Pauline criterion of an "apostle," that is, she was sent by the risen Jesus to preach the gospel.[2] Despite some subordinationist texts in the Pauline corpus (possibly later insertions), Paul writes to women as leaders of the churches he founded and includes them in central positions in his ministry. His keynote—from which he occasionally wavers—is "There is neither Jew nor Greek, there is neither slave nor free, there is neither male nor female; for you are all one in Christ Jesus" (Gal. 3:28).[3]

In neither the Hebrew tradition nor early Christianity is the morality of sexual conduct a major or independent interest. Sexuality, marriage, and family relations are always seen in relation to the nature and vocation of the people of God, and to the sort of faith and obedience that should characterize its members. There is no specific development of a "sexual ethics" in the New Testament.[4] The only extended treatment of marriage occurs in 1 Corinthians 7. The purpose of marriage on which Paul focuses there is the legitimate satisfaction of sexual passion (vv. 2, 9, 36–37). Procreation is not a particular objective of the Christian community; Paul explicitly anticipates the end of the world and the fulfillment of the reign of God in the near future (vv. 26, 29, 31b). As far as he is concerned, marriage and the obligations it entails only distract from preparation for the kingdom (vv. 32–35). However, within the state of marriage, husband and wife are equal participants and are viewed as equally obligated in the things that concern marriage (vv. 2–4, 10–14, 16, 32–34). Another striking dissimilarity to the Hebrew view of sexuality is Paul's preference for virginity over the married state (vv. 7–8, 38–40). As in the Hebrew tradition, Paul gauges human activity by its contribution to the community of faith (1 Cor. 12–14). However, in light of his eschatological expectations, he concludes that the single state better facilitates "undivided devotion to the Lord" (v. 35).

Paul does acknowledge that even though not all can live as celibates, "each has his own special gift from God, one of one kind and one of another" (v. 7), and suggests that the faith of a married believer can "consecrate" his or her spouse and children (v. 14). This hints at the potential contributions of the married state to the Christian community. Yet on the whole Paul sees neither marriage nor parenthood as positive Christian callings. Similarly, sexual activity is not seen as good for its own sake nor as a positive means to worthwhile goals such as mutual love and procreation. Rather it is something that is permissible for those who need it, provided that it is kept in the proper context.

The five sayings on divorce that occur in the New Testament (Lk. 16:18; Mk. 10:1–12; Mt. 5:32 and 19:9, and 1 Cor. 7:10–11) demonstrate both the inviolability of the marriage bond and the priority given by New Testament authors to the communal life of discipleship as the framework within which morality is to be evaluated. Faithful life in community takes precedence over moral laws as such, and even over the normative function of isolated sayings of Jesus. While it is relatively certain that Jesus himself prohibited divorce (by Paul's explicit testimony, 1 Cor. 7:10–11), faith communities familiar with his teaching confronted the task of making his sayings relevant to their own life situations. Not all applications and exceptions could have been contemplated by Jesus or contained in the original dictum. Thus Matthew adds that divorce is wrong "except for *porneia*" (unchastity) (5:32; 19:9), and Paul makes an exception for the sake of "peace" for Christian converts married to unwilling nonbelievers (1 Cor. 7:15). Scholars remain uncertain as to the precise meanings of these exceptive qualifications, and even as to whether they constitute exceptions in the usual sense of the word.[5] It is clear, however, that the New Testament itself provides a model for the continuing interpretive appropriation of authoritative teaching within the historical faith community.

Absent both in the New Testament and in the early Church is any positive appreciation of sexual intercourse, even in the light of married love and parenthood. This is in striking contrast to the Old Testament, especially the Song of Songs. One reason for the more negative interpretation of sexuality in the first century after Christ may be the influence of the Greek and Roman Stoic philosophies that were a part of contemporary culture. The Stoics aimed to gain control over human existence, and escape the unhappiness that arises from its contingencies, by subordinating all emotions and passions to rational ends, or even to rise above passion completely. Obviously, the denigration of passion puts sexuality in a dubious light. This influence already appears to be present in the writings of St. Paul and continues into the patristic period. For the Stoics, the sole justification of sexual acts becomes the rationally commendable goal of procreation. As primitive Christianity moved toward the second generation it appropriated Stoic themes while trying simultaneously to counteract some views encountered in Hellenistic Gnosticism—for instance, that the material world is evil, that the body imprisons the soul, and that procreation is wrong because it perpetuates captivity of souls.

CHRISTIAN TRADITION

Drawing on the Hebrew tradition of a good Creator of the world and of humanity, the first generations of Christians affirmed the goodness of the body as well as the soul, and thus approved sex, marriage, and bearing children. Yet, with Stoicism, there was a tendency to see freedom from passion as preferable to and higher than even a moderate experience of it, and to set procreation as the rationally defined end that best justifies sexual acts.

Early views of the goodness of the married state and of parenthood seem to vary in inverse proportion to the urgency of eschatological expectation. A celibate life for all believers may seem feasible in the short term, but as the end time is delayed, institutions that preserve human life in the meantime appear as good and necessary. The Latin Father Tertullian (c. 160–c. 225), who anticipated an imminent Second Coming, exalted virginity and even exhorted spouses to aim for the celibate ideal. An extreme form of this rigorously ascetic strain of Christianity was Montanism, which held that the world was about to end, that all believers ideally should be celibate, and that there was no forgiveness of sins committed after baptism. Although Montanism was eventually rejected as heretical by the Church, Tertullian increasingly identified himself with it, so that later in his life he not only counseled virginity but also spoke of all second marriage as adultery.[6] Clement of Alexandria (c. 150–c. 215) was a Greek contemporary of Tertullian who was sympathetic to Stoic ideals but incorporated them more moderately into Christianity. Clement agreed that continence is better than sexual relations, but much more decisively affirms the institution of marriage by God as part of the creation and thus as a commendable state.[7]

One great figure in the patristic period makes the most significant contribution to subsequent Christian views of sexuality and marriage and sets the parameters of future discussion both for medieval Christianity and for Reformation Christianity. This theologian is Augustine (354–430), Bishop of Hippo in North Africa, then a Roman province. Augustine's contribution is both positive and negative, if the standard is appreciation of the value of sex, marriage, and parenthood. Certainly Augustine follows the biblical and Church tradition that human life and the means necessary to continue it are created good. Yet the corruption by sin of everything human leaves a vast intellectual and, evidently, emotional impression on Augustine. One can speculate on the origins of his fascination with the sinful possibilities of sexuality when one reads his own accounts of his life with a faithful concubine, whom he abandoned after fifteen years at his mother's behest, taking with him their son.[8] An ambivalence about sexuality is reflected in Augustine's theology and ethics. He seems disturbed by the prospect that any aspect of human conduct should escape full control by the reason and will. Like the Stoics, Augustine believed that the rational faculty ought to dominate the passions and control the body. A disordered love, or "concupiscence," is one in which the will is deflected from its proper object, God, and the ordering of all else in relation to God.[9] Of necessity, intercourse is not fully under the control of the rational will but, especially for the male, involves a physical response that an intellectual decision is not sufficient to evoke. Thus, Augustine seems convinced that in the actual order of things, after the Fall, sexual intercourse always is tainted by sin, and may even be the means by which original sin is transmitted to offspring.[10]

Although Augustine too saw virginity as higher than sexual activity even in marriage,[11] he countered the dualistic Manichean doctrine that matter is created by an evil power by defining the purpose of sexual union as procreation. Marriage, the context of legitimate sexual activity, has three purposes: children *(proles)*, fidelity and the avoidance of fornication *(fides)*, and the indissoluble and sacramental bond of Christian spouses *(sacramentum)*,[12] which symbolizes the love of Christ for the Church.[13] Augustine also speaks of the companionship with which men and women provide one another,[14] though mutual love is not given as one of the primary goods of the marriage union, much less of sexual expression. More definitively than in any other author, the Christian tradition in Augustine sets parenthood as the agenda of the sexual life, and establishes the marriage of one man and one women as the framework within which this agenda is to be fulfilled.

The benchmark of Catholic theology and ethics is the theological synthesis of Thomas Aquinas (1224/5–1274), who intertwined Christian teaching and Aristotelian philosophy with originality and imagination, claiming all the while the authorities of the tradition as his foundation. Not least among these is Augustine, from whom Aquinas takes many specific references to the moral life, including the goods of marriage. The distinctive flavor of Aquinas's treatment, however, derives from his Christian interpretation of Aristotle's premise that the world consists in a hierarchy of beings with distinct "natures" or intrinsic principles of existence and activity. The unique marks of human nature are rationality and free will. These capacities combine with the underlying physical structure of the human person to provide the criteria of moral responsibility. Human moral activity is to be rational, free, and respectful of the natural needs and the purposes of the human body. This perspective constitutes the basis of the "natural-law" approach to ethics. In a fundamental way it is an empirical approach. Human experience reveals what is most fulfilling for humans. Reason and intelligence are needed to interpret experience, however, in order to distinguish what is *essentially* "natural" (morally appropriate) human conduct, as differentiated from behavior that humans may often exhibit, but which is not in conformity with their true nature or highest ideals.

The natural-law view of ethics is essentially optimistic. While it recognizes the impediments of sin, it places a great deal of confidence in human ability to know and do that which is most consistent with authentic human values and human welfare. Scripture and the authority of the Church clarify these values and hold them up for emulation, but do not contribute anything which is not in principle evident to any reasonable and well-intentioned moral agent. A perduring problem for the Catholic natural-law tradition of ethics has been to define precisely how it is that "natural" human values can be known and taught clearly, given the fact that values must always be perceived from within a particular set of historical circumstances; and the fact that "reason" always means the intellects of individuals or groups of individuals, who must cooperate in generalizing about the values known from experience. As Aquinas himself cautioned, the "practical reason . . . is busied with contingent matters, about which human actions are concerned: and consequently, although there is necessity in the general principles the more we descend to matters of detail, the more we encounter defects." Thus, "as to the proper conclusions of the practical reason, neither is the truth or rectitude the same for all, nor, where it is the same, is it equally known by all."[15] In other words, it is not so difficult for human beings to agree at a general level, by affirming, for instance, the importance of respect for life or procreation of the species—but exactly *when* it is legitimate to take a human life, or exactly *how* children are to be born and educated may be less certain, and will be subject to discussion and argument.

The magisterium or "teaching authority" of the Catholic Church has as one of its functions to guide human reason in the process of thinking through the concrete meanings of generally acknowledged human values in important areas of human activity. It claims this function by virtue of the presence of the Holy Spirit within the Church as the people of God or Body of Christ. Even so, not all problems are resolved. What relation does authoritative religious guidance have to reasonable argument? Does the validity of the magisterium's teachings depend on the persuasive power of the arguments offered on their behalf? If not, then exactly who is it to whom the Church speaks, and what becomes of the fundamental "natural-law" commitment to a community of moral discourse?

Aquinas's view of sexual morality depends both on Christian religious teaching and on his understanding of what is natural to humans. His view is informed by the traditional enumeration of the "three goods," mediated to him from Augustine via the *Sentences* of Peter Lombard.[16] But Aquinas thinks that the tradition can be defended as reasonable and self-evident apart from authority. Another important source is the Roman jurist Ulpian, who emphasized the moral implications of those aspects of human nature that are shared with other animals, for instance the procreative design of copulation. Aquinas continues the common tradition that permanent, monogamous, procreative, and patriarchal marriage realizes the essentially natural and hence normative meaning of sexual acts and relations. At the same time, he expands and revises Augustine's moral perspective on sex and marriage. Aquinas nowhere suggests that passion or sexual desire is intrinsically suspect, or need override the ends of human activity prescribed by nature. Even more importantly for the development of a view of sex as contributing to and expressing the interpersonal spousal relationship, Aquinas calls attention to the friendship and love that should exist in marriage, and which is intensified by sexual intercourse.[17] Sex is primarily "for" procreation, but occurs in a relation also characterized by a strong and appropriate affective bond and commitment.

The stress on the mutual friendship that should characterize marriage also helps counteract the subordinationist view of women which Aquinas preserves both from Aristotle and from Augustine, and which goes more or less unchallenged in his writings.[18] Aquinas does recognize that both men and women belong to the perfection of the species,[19] and that both sexes were created by God out of preexisting material, which God "formed immediately" into a human being.[20] He also takes note that the Genesis creation stories do not substantiate any "servile" role for wives,[21] even if women are naturally less rational, physically weaker, and so subordinate, and to be ruled even in the domestic relationship by the husband.

Monogamy and indissolubility are naturally required in marriage by the duty to raise up offspring, and in respect of the friendship of the spouses, but for Christians, the permanence of marriage is also a sign of Christ's presence to the

Church.[22] The articulation of the meaning of Christian marriage in the language of "sacrament" is a means of conferring upon it a positive value in relation to the community that it does not have in the New Testament. A biblical text often used as a basis of the sacramental meaning of marriage is Ephesians 5, where husbands are exhorted to "love your wives, as Christ loved the church" (v. 25), and where Paul comments of the "mystery" of the "one flesh" unity of wife and husband that "I am saying that it refers to Christ and the church" (v. 32). Certainly there is here no developed theology of sacrament as a sign that makes present the reality signified. Taken on its own terms, the reference to the love of Christ for Church may only go so far as an example of what faithful love is like, not as far as an assertion that married love actually participates in the love Christ bears toward the Christian community. It is important, however, that an appreciation of the natural meaning of marriage led theologians and Church teachers to place it in the sphere of the revelation of God's loving faithfulness toward humanity. Marriage was listed formally as a sacrament of the Church—along with baptism, confession, and eucharist—at the Council of Verona (1184), in response to a revival of the dualism against which patristic authors, preeminently Augustine, had fought.[23]

During the Reformation of the sixteenth century, leaders such as Luther and Calvin disputed the sacramental and indissoluble status of marriage. This was not primarily because they regarded it as an inferior state, but because they wanted to loosen ecclesiasical control over a relation which they considered good and worthy but essentially secular. Institutional corruptions of medieval Christianity led them to limit the sphere in which Church authority could operate. In response, the Council of Trent reasserted in the decree *Tametsi* that Christian marriage is permanent, is a sacrament, and moreover requires a specified form in order to be valid; it must be celebrated in the presence of a priest and two witnesses.

"After *Tametsi*, as before, the sacrament of marriage is still constituted by the consent of the man and the woman, and the marriage is constituted indissoluble by their subsequent intercourse."[24]

These provisions became incorporated in the canon law of the Roman Church and have contributed to the Roman Catholic perspective on the nature of the marriage bond. Positively, it is a commendable human relationship in which grace is communicated and which serves as a sign of grace to the Christian community. Within this context, designed for and completed by the sexual expression of love and commitment, children are born and nurtured. Negatively, Church teaching did not retract the second-class status of marriage in relation to the vowed religious life, a status about which the Reformers were at least skeptical. By assigning marriage to a juridical context, the Church contributed to a legalistic and contractarian view of the privileges and obligations of spouses. The 1917 Code of Canon Law also gave impetus to the idea that procreation should be a primary goal of spouses, by relegating mutual help and "remedy for concupiscence" to secondary status.[25]

Through the patristic, medieval, Reformation, and post-Reformation periods, then, there have developed central standards for sexual expression, which link it with marriage as a context and parenthood as an outcome. Celibacy is more highly valued but is not mandatory; sexual acts are justified completely only by the intention of procreation; they should be carried out in a heterosexual, monogamous, and permanent relationship. To seek intercourse with one's spouse for physical release or pleasure is not commendable but is tolerated (as a "venial" sin); the petitioned spouse is enjoined to comply, that is, to "render the debt" (cf. 1 Cor. 7:3–4). The possibility that marriage is first and foremost an interpersonal love relationship is virtually ignored; indeed, it may have been a barely imaginable idea before the Enlightenment and Reformation emphasis on the individual and on the importance of individual commitment. Before that time, marriage was a form of social and kinship organization from which individuals derived both their social and their personal roles, not, as today, a public expression of roles that individuals freely choose to assume and whose meaning is created largely out of their love for each other.

Post-Enlightenment Western Christianity has stressed the value and subjective experience of the individual and has put the importance of the individual person on a par with that of social groups. There have been significant consequences in our views of the morality of sexual relationships, and of the meanings of marriage and parenthood, even when considered as institutions with a social dimension. Personal fulfillment and the quality of interpersonal relationship have risen in importance as the standards of sexual union and of all relationships within the family. It is precisely these criteria that motivate questions about the absolute unbreakability of the sexual and emotional bond of husband and wife, about the reasons for becoming a parent and the morally available means of avoiding or accomplishing pregnancy and birth, and about the importance of confining sex to a monogamous, heterosexual union appropriate for raising children.

MODERN ROMAN CATHOLICISM

As recently as 1930, Pope Pius XI, in his encyclical letter *Casti Connubii*, cites the authority of Augustine in defending procreation as the primary purpose of marriage.

> The saintly Doctor shows that the whole doctrine of Christian wedlock is excellently summarized under these three heads: '*Fidelity* signifies that outside the matrimonial bond there shall be no sexual intercourse; *Offspring* sig-

nifies that children shall be lovingly welcomed, tenderly reared, and religiously educated; *Sacrament* signifies that the bond of wedlock shall never be broken, and that neither party, if separated, shall form a union with another, even for the sake of offspring. Such is the law of marriage, which gives luster to the fruitfulness of nature and sets a curb upon shameful incontinence.' . . . Among the blessings of marriage offspring holds the first place.[26]

The Pope also upholds the indissolubility of Christian marriage and the proper submission of wife to husband. He excludes birth control from marital sexuality by stating that "The conjugal act is of its very nature designed for the procreation of offspring; and therefore those who in performing it deliberately deprive it of its natural power and efficacy, act against nature and do something which is shameful and intrinsically immoral."[27]

Without specifically rejecting past teaching, the Second Vatican Council document *Gaudium et Spes* assumes a strikingly different tone in speaking of married love and its relation to procreation. First of all, conjugal love involves "the good of the whole person" and is expressed appropriately in "the marital act" that is "noble and worthy" and which signifies and promotes "the mutual self-giving" of spouses.[28] "Marriage and conjugal love are by their nature ordained toward the begetting and educating of children." However, marriage "to be sure is not instituted solely for procreation," but must also embody "the mutual love of spouses," since "marriage persists as a whole manner and communion of life."[29] *Gaudium et Spes* does not specifically mention contraception—shortly to be addressed independently by the Pope[30]—but does outline the framework within which such questions of sexual morality are to be undertaken:

Therefore when there is question of harmonizing conjugal love with the responsible transmission of life, the moral aspect of any procedure does not depend solely on sincere intentions or on an evaluation of motives. It must be determined by objective standards. These, based on the nature of the human person and his acts, preserve the full sense of mutual self-giving and human procreation in the context of true love.[31]

Also the teaching authority of the Church must be respected in this regard, since the Church is charged with the "unfolding of the divine law."

A clarifying statement on artificial birth control was provided by Paul VI in the encyclical *Humanae Vitae* (1968). After the death of John XXIII, Paul expanded the papal commission on birth control that his predecessor had convened, and it was Paul to whom the commission eventually submitted its recommendations. A majority of commission members was convinced that a procreative purpose expressed over the entirety of a marriage and its sexual acts was adequate to the unity of marital love and parenthood. However, Paul adopted as the foundation of his own position the opinion of the minority that each marital sexual act must be open to the possibility of procreation—that is, must be not artificially prevented from achieving that end.[32] Yet it is permissible to take advantage of the natural rhythms of fecundity. "Nonetheless, the Church, calling men back to the observance of the norms of the natural law, as interpreted by her constant doctrine, teaches that each and every marriage act must remain open to the transmission of life."[33] It is an error to suppose that a sexual act "which is deliberately made infecund and so is intrinsically dishonest could be made honest and right by the ensemble of a fecund conjugal life."[34]

Attention to the encyclical's close delimitation of sexuality in marriage should not be permitted to obscure the significant progress in the Catholic understanding of marriage that is also represented by the encyclical. Most importantly, procreation is not presented as the primary purpose of marriage or of sex. The "two great realities of married life" are "conjugal love" on the one hand and, on the other, not procreation as such but "responsible parenthood."[35] Like *Gaudium et Spes*, *Humanae Vitae* speaks of marital love in terms of "communion" and "reciprocal personal gift of self"[36] and, like Aquinas, as "a very special form of personal friendship."[37] Finally, *Humanae Vitae* warns not only of the violation of the intrinsic nature of love and sex that contraception is said to pose, but also of consequent dangers to human attitudes toward conception and parenthood that technology may present. "[I]f the mission of generating life is not to be exposed to the arbitrary will of men, one must necessarily recognize insurmountable limits to the possibility of man's domination over his own body and its functions," limits that "cannot be determined otherwise than by the respect due to the integrity of the human organism and its functions."[38] Hardly anywhere in recent Church teaching is found more evident the tensive and often elusive interplay between reasonable arguments about what is fitting to human "nature" and arguments about what is consistent with past Church teaching, whether or not that Church teaching continues to appear reasonable. Ambiguity about the sense and authority of teaching in the case of sexual morality derives in great part from the shift in Church understanding of the marital relationship that has been occurring at least since Vatican II, but which has not been accompanied by a commensurate shift in Catholic understanding of the morality of the acts which express that relationship. This difficulty continues to be pronounced in the writings of the present Pope, John Paul II.

John Paul brings three distinctive emphases to his considerations of sexuality, marriage, and parenthood that are not evident as strongly in previous Catholic teaching. These emphases reflect developments in Catholic moral theology generally since Vatican II. First, he makes a concentrated effort to ground his reflections in appropriate biblical accounts of the meaning and destiny of human life; second, he articulates his philosophical and experiential understandings of human "nature" in the language of twentieth-century "personalist" philosophy; third, he portrays women and men as equal partners in marriage and family. At the level of specific sexual morality within marriage, he retains the conclusion of previous Popes that both love and procreation are inseparable purposes of each and every sexual act, and that this is required by the vary natures of human sexuality and of conjugal love. The three fundamental emphases are much in evidence in John Paul's series of audience talks on the "Theology of the Body" (1979–1981).[39] A favorite phrase, "the nuptial meaning of the body," is offered as a commentary on Adam's recognition of the woman, "This at last is bone of my bone and flesh of my flesh." That exclamation confirms "the reciprocity and communion of persons" which sexual difference makes possible, and which is established in the conjugal "one flesh" unity. The body's "nuptial meaning" as revealed in these texts consists preeminently in the fact that "a creature God willed for its own sake . . . can fully discover its true self only in a sincere giving of self."[40] Moreover, the blessing of increase of Genesis 1 is combined with the conjugal theme of Genesis 2, so that John Paul can say that "the spouses-parents" unite "so closely as to become 'one flesh' " and so "subject, in a way, their humanity to the blessing of fertility, namely, 'procreation,' of which the first narrative speaks (Gen. 1:28)."[41]

Sexual expression becomes "the language of the body" in a true "communion of persons." Truthful sexual acts must signify not only love but also "potential fecundity," as has been taught by *Humanae Vitae*. Thus "the conjugal act, deprived of its interior truth because deprived of its procreative capacity, ceases also to be an act of love."[42] Similarly, in his apostolic exhortation "On the Family" *(Familiaris Consortio)*, John Paul responds to the 1980 Synod on the family with similar personalist and biblical themes, and in support of the same concrete conclusion about sexual acts. All sex acts are to occur in marriage and are to be open to procreation: this is demanded by the nature of conjugal love itself. The "unitive" and "procreative" meanings of the "conjugal act" are "inseparable."

> When couples, by means of recourse to contraception, separate these two meanings that God the Creator has inscribed in the being of man and woman and in the dynamism of sexual communion, they act as 'arbiters' of the divine plan and they 'manipulate' and degrade human sexuality and with it themselves and their married partner by altering its value of 'total' self-giving.[43]

Positive contributions here are the efforts to take biblical resources seriously as a foundation of moral understanding and to link moral teaching about sex and parenthood with the concrete experience of married love. The physical and interpersonal aspects of sexuality are woven into one approach; and morality is based on both rather than primarily on the physical structure of the reproductive processes. Men and women contribute equally to marriage, love, and parenthood. This equality is confirmed in those passages of *Familiaris Consortio* in which John Paul affirms both the roles of women in public functions in society and of men as husbands and fathers in the home (even though the parental role seems still to be associated somewhat more closely with the true nature of women).[44] However, once the legitimacy of roles of women beyond parenthood is affirmed equally with those of men; once the experiential source of reflection on the "nature" of marital sexuality is the interpersonal love relationship over and above the physical procreative process; and once the ultimate criterion is the Genesis creation stories, which do not focus on individual acts, as did traditional Catholic moral theology—then does the integrity of the natural process of sexual intercourse, conception, and birth still survive as a decisive mandate in defining the moral obligations of marital, parental sexuality?

In his classic work, *Contraception,* John T. Noonan attempts to enlarge the sphere of reference of the Church's condemnation of contraception by highlighting several "core" values which that prohibition represents, but which may not necessarily be tied to its perpetuation precisely in its current, magisterial form. The key propositions that the prohibition protects are: "Procreation is good. Procreation of offspring reaches its completion only in their education. Innocent life is sacred. The personal dignity of a spouse is to be respected. Marital love is holy."[45] But these values of procreation, education, life, personality, and love were protected by means of a specific doctrine against contraceptive acts that took shape in combat with historical influences hostile to all procreation (Gnosticism, Manicheeism, Catharism). It was "molded by the teaching of the Gospels on the sanctity of marriage; the Pauline condemnation of unnatural sexual behavior; the Old Testament emphasis on fertility; the desire to justify marriage while extolling virginity; the need to assign rational purpose and limit to sexual behavior. The doctrine was formed in a society where slavery, slave concubinage, and the inferiority of women were important elements of the environment affecting sexual relations. The education of children was neither universal nor expensive. Underpopulation was a main governmental concern." Asks Noonan, "Was the commitment to an absolute prohibition of contraception more conscious, more universal, more complete, than to . . . now obsolete rules" against intercourse in menstruation, intercourse in pregnancy, and intercourse in other than the "natural" position?[46] Noonan's rhetorical questions suggest, of course, that it was not, but that the specific formulation of the teaching protected the five core values in ways that were appropriate to particular historical contexts with their peculiar threats and opportunities. A new formulation may be vital to the survival of the same values in changed circumstances, which pose new questions about the concrete meaning of respect for those values.

Ambiguity in the development of Catholic tradition about the meaning and morality of sexuality, marriage, and parenthood is also reflected in canon law, especially in the 1983 revision of the 1917 Code, in light of the themes of Vatican II. Several theologians and canonists have suggested that the 1983 Code only partially realizes the insights of the Council,[47] with the result that the latter's view of marriage as a "partnership of the whole of life"[48] is not permitted to influence fully the juridical treatment of marriage, its constituent elements, and its obligations. Thus in many ways, marriage is still regarded as a "contract" in which each party freely and hence irrevocably consents to yield to the other an exclusive right to his or her body regarding acts by nature directed to procreation.[49] The canonist Ladislas Orsy observes,

> The new Code has retained the strongly institutional orientation of the old one but the insights of the Council concerning the dignity and rights of individual persons have made substantial inroads into the old structures. The result is a somewhat uneasy coexistence of two diverging trends, one upholding the primacy of the institution, the other the importance of human persons. Also, the understanding of marriage appears now in a broad religious context through the doctrine of the covenant, yet the highly juridical language of the contract is still present in many traditionally formulated canons.[50]

The problem in the canonical approach is essentially the same as in the ethical approach. The Church's understanding of the reality in question has shifted from an individualistic and act-centered focus to an appreciation of the continuous and self-involving reciprocal relationship that constitutes marriage and is the context for understanding acts. In the case of canon law, the preeminent "acts" are the acts of consent and of consummation; in the case of moral theology, the "acts" are sexual intercourse and conception. In both cases, the acts remain the focus of the formulation of specific norms (for defining indissolubility on the one hand, and for defining sexual morality on the other), even after the Church has accepted some fundamental changes in understanding the relationship underlying the acts, and has come to see that it is not after all the acts that are the prism through which to comprehend the relationship, but the other way around.

REFLECTIONS

As it entered the second half of the twentieth century, the Roman Catholic tradition on sexuality, marriage, and parenthood arrived with an internal inconsistency. In the first place, the love of spouses was seen increasingly as a good of marriage, and a purpose of their sexual relationship with an importance equal to that of procreation. It even is arguable that in many respects love is not only equal but primary as a meaning of marriage in the context of which to understand sexual morality. The writings of John Paul II are not inhospitable to such an interpretation when they affirm the mutual self-gift of wife and husband as the meaning of marriage and the reality that sexual acts are to express. The Pope even bases his natural law prohibition of contraception on the same basis: the intrinsic meaning of marital *love*. The crucial importance of loving commitment in canonical approaches to defining marriage is reflected in those aspects of the 1983 Code which build on the insight of *Gaudium et Spes* that marriage is a partnership of the whole of life, not just a mutual agreement to the *jus in corpus* of the 1917 Code. In the second place, however, those norms prescribing the morality of sexual and procreative acts that are affirmed currently by the teaching authority of the Church, are the same norms that were originally derived from the more act-focused and often individualist understanding of sexuality. Further, this older model often delineates human sexual "nature" in terms of physical nature (the integrity of the reproductive process), so that moral norms regarding sexuality are grounded primarily in that structure, rather than on the interpersonal meanings of sexual acts in relation to marital and parental love.

This ambiguity has significant consequences for the Catholic ethics of sex, parenthood, and marriage. Most fundamentally, there is a less than adequate Christian respect for the integrity of body and soul, in which both are valued together and together form an object of moral reflection, but in which there is also a recognition that it is the intellect and will (and affections) which are distinctively human. We have seen that in the premodern tradition, traces of dualism survived Augustine's affirmation of the goodness of the material world, so that the body was viewed not only as an inferior component of the human person, but even as an occasion of sin to be suppressed. Procreation was offered as the justification of physical sexual desire and acts, and it was the physical structure of those acts that determined their essential morality. Once sexual morality is tied decisively to the physical components of sexual acts, it becomes difficult to make exceptions to the norms so derived, even to serve the personal good of spouses, children, or families.

On the other hand, the hidden presuppositions of modern Western sexual mores are also problematic, and for some of the same reasons. For all the modern exaltation of the body and the goodness of sexuality, our views of sex are too often premised on a dualism in which the body is really seen as inferior. Free consent at the minimum, or love at the maximum, becomes the sovereign norm of sexual conduct. Physical conditions or consequences of sexual conduct, such as conception and birth, cease to function as morally normative at all. The writings of John Paul II, to the extent that they romanticize and idealize the interpersonal love relationship, while grounding substantive norms in the physical act, continue to discourage the true integration of spirit and body as sources of sexual ethics. What is needed is a sexual ethics that recognizes both the physical and interpersonal aspects of sexuality, marriage, and parenthood. Moreover, the goal of an integrated view of sex, love, and procreation will not be achieved until due attention is accorded to the broader economic and social settings in which these relationships have their concrete existence. Factors such as patriarchal or egalitarian gender roles, the relation of the family to the larger social order, and available economic resources for couples and their children can have bearing on what is right or wrong, just or unjust, prudent or destructive for persons to undertake in their sexual lives.

If norms are to be set for and limits to be put on sexual morality, what should they be? The overriding moral criterion should be an interpersonal one: love, especially the committed love commensurate with full sexual expression. "Love" in this case may include an affective, emotional attachment, but it primarily signifies a commitment to create with one's spouse a cooperative partnership in sexuality, parenthood, and in the domestic and social roles that pertain to the couple and the family. The centrality of love as a norm in sexual morality is consistent with the personal character of the "one-flesh" union of Adam and Eve, with Jesus' emphasis on the involvement of one's deepest attitudes and commitments in one's moral activity, with the Thomistic tradition's stress on distinctively human characteristics as most important to human "nature" and as essential to "friendship," with the post-Vatican II teaching on marriage as a personal relationship of commitment, and with John Paul II's view of sex as the language of mutual self-gift.

To stipulate that the special context of love that sex and parenthood require is a marital commitment gives recognition to the physical or material sphere as well as to the interpersonal one. Marriage is a form of social participation that gives access to the social goods necessary for the nurturing of children and for the support so crucial to the stability and longevity of a love relationship. This is not to short-circuit discussion about whether the Western, contractual understanding of marriage is adequate, especially from a Christian perspective. More consideration should be given to the possibility that marriage is a process undertaken gradually, neither beginning suddenly with the public exchange of vows, nor after that time complete and irrevocable. However, within the trinity of love, sex, and procreation, it is love that is fundamental, most humanly distinctive, and thus most morally important. Sex and procreation are not merely dispensable goods, but their moral meaning can be defined fully only within the interpersonal relationship of the persons who cooperate in realizing these goods.

3.

An Overview of the Instruction

The purpose of this chapter is to give an overview of the structure, teaching, and implications of the recent Vatican statement on human life and procreation. This will help situate both the substance of the teaching and provide the basis for a more detailed evaluation elsewhere in the book. Here we simply identify the major themes and issues of the document.

The "Instruction on Respect for Human Life in Its Origin and on the Dignity of Procreation" was issued by the Congregation for the Doctrine of the Faith on 22 February 1987. Cardinal Joseph Ratzinger signed the document and it was released with the approval of Pope John Paul II. According to the foreword, the document is a response to inquiries from episcopal conferences, individual bishops, theologians, doctors, and scientists about the liceity of interventions into human reproduction. This instruction, which is the "result of wide consultation and in particular of the declarations made by episcopates,"[1] provides a response to these queries.

The introduction sets the general context and tone of the document by focusing on the place and role of technology within the human community. Here fundamental criteria are set forth. Chapter 1 discusses the human embryo. After establishing the respect due to it, the instruction then discusses prenatal diagnosis, research and experimentation, and other manipulations of the human embryo. Chapter 2 discusses interventions in human reproduction. Heterologous and homologous artificial fertilization are discussed, both with respect to IVF and artificial insemination. The document also takes note of the problems and sufferings caused by the experience of infertility. Chapter 3 focuses on moral and civil law and identifies the values that ought to stand behind any civil legislation affecting human reproduction. The document concludes with an exhortation to continue the moral and scientific study of human reproduction, but within the context of respect for human dignity and the moral values derived from that.

MORAL CRITERIA USED IN THE ANALYSIS

In general, the document argues its case in terms of the traditional natural-law teaching of the Catholic Church, amplified by revelation and mediated through papal and magisterial teaching. The expression of this teaching follows some of the orientation initiated by Vatican II with its emphasis on the person and the language of rights. This orientation has been continued by John Paul II in his encyclicals and speeches.[2]

1. Morality and Science

The document argues that the meaning of science and technology must be drawn from the nature of the person and his or her moral values. Thus science and technology are valuable when they promote "his integral development for the benefit of all,"[3] And very importantly the document notes a point frequently missed by many: "They [science and technology] cannot of themselves show the meaning of existence and of human progress."[4] Science is a method and as a method it helps us achieve certain ends, but the method itself cannot evaluate those ends. By implication, then, the instruction rejects the technological imperative that says that if we can do something, we must. The point of departure, then, is science at the service of humans. This point is affirmed toward the end of the document:

> Medicine which seeks to be ordered to the integral good of the person must respect the specifically human values of sexuality. The doctor is at the service of persons and of human procreation. He does not have the authority to dispose of them or to decide their fate.[5]

Thus there is an inherent check on science and technology: the nature of the person.

2. Respect for Human Persons

The key value in the instruction is respect for the dignity of the human person. The criteria for evaluating interventions are

> the respect, defense and promotion of man, his 'primary and fundamental right' to life, his dignity as a person who is endowed with a spiritual soul and with moral responsibility and who is called to beatific communion with God.[6]

This dignity extends also to the physical life of an individual. While this physical dimension does not ". . . contain the whole of a person's value, nor does it represent the supreme good of man," physical life constitutes a fundamental value because upon it ". . . all the other values of the person are based and developed."[7] The instruction also specifies the extent of that respect by noting: "The human being must be respected—as a person—from the very first instant of his existence."[8] This also ensures that the person at any time during his or her existence must not be exploited. Thus to create a life simply for the purpose of using it as research material is immoral.[9]

The relation between the physical and transcendent dimension of the person is based on the claim that

> An intervention on the human body affects not only the tissues, the organs and their functions, but also involves the person himself on different levels.[10]

Because of the holistic nature of the person—his or her psychosomatic unity—there is no such thing as a merely technical intervention. Insofar as the interventions are purposeful and performed on the human, they have an inescapable moral dimension. Thus the concept of respect for persons, both physically and spiritually, stands as the touchstone of the moral analysis of the reproductive technologies.

3. Avoidance of Harms

A concept familiar to most bioethicists is that of nonmalfeasance, the obligation to avoid harm. The instruction uses this concept as another curb on artificial interventions. Thus, in discussing both prenatal diagnosis and experimentation on the fetus, the duty not to harm plays a critical role. Interventions are possible only if they respect the life of the embryo and the mother and do not subject them "to disproportionate risks."[11] This often-used term is defined in the instruction with respect to evaluating "possible negative consequences" that may be the byproduct of a necessary use of a particular technique. Such techniques should be avoided if they do "not offer sufficient guarantees of their honest purpose and substantial harmlessness."[12] Thus the document recognizes that various interventions might be proposed, but one needs to test them by considering whether or not they are "directed to the pure promotion of the personal well-being of the individual without doing harm to his integrity or worsening his conditions of life."[13]

4. Rights

Two rights are considered in the instruction, one which is positively asserted and one whose reality is denied. The positive right is the right of a child

> to be conceived, carried in the womb, brought into the world and brought up within marriage. . ."[14]

This right secures the identity of the child and promotes the achievement of his or her own development.

The invalidity of another right is discussed within the context of infertility.

> Nevertheless, marriage does not confer upon the spouses the right to have a child, but only the right to perform those natural acts which are per se ordered to procreation.[15]

If there were to be a right to a child, the child's dignity and nature would be violated by it. The child is "not an object to which one has a right nor can he be considered as an object of ownership."[16] Rather, the child is a gift, a gift of marriage and a testimony to the mutual giving of the parents. An entitlement to a child would, in the judgment of the instruction destroy the graciousness of the reality of the child.

5. Fidelity of the Spouses

A traditional good of marriage, the fidelity of the spouses, serves here as a critical moral value. First, the fidelity of the spouses involves "reciprocal respect of their right to become a father and a mother only through each other."[17] Second, such fidelity makes possible the procreation of the child "in conformity with the dignity of the person."[18] Third, the fidelity of the spouses reflects the twofold structure of the conjugal act: the unitive and the procreative. Maintaining the inseparability of these dimensions prevents the violation of marriage through introducing a third party, preserves the child's relation with his or her parents, and maintains true mutual love and the vocation to parenthood. Consequently,

> In order to respect the language of their bodies and their natural generosity, the conjugal union must take place with respect for its openness to procreation; and the procreation of a person must be the fruit and the result of married love. The origin of the human being thus follows from a procreation that is 'linked to the union, not only biological but also spiritual, of the parents, made one by the bond of marriage.' Fertilization achieved outside the bodies of the couple remains by this very fact deprived of the meanings and the values which are expressed in the language of the body and in the union of human persons.[19]

Summary

These five moral values or principles are the foundation on the basis of which various reproductive technologies are evaluated. The principles are clearly identified from within the Catholic Christian tradition of natural law and magisterial teaching, and give rise to unavoidable duties. We now turn to the application of these principles.

APPLICATION OF PRINCIPLES

Five specific issues are addressed in the instruction with other possibilities being commented on by inference. The instruction applies the principles described above as the basis for decision making.

1. Prenatal Diagnosis

Prenatal diagnosis permits the health status of the fetus to be evaluated. Thus it can help treatment begin earlier, can prepare the parents and health-care providers for the needs of the baby, and it can be the basis on which individuals request an abortion. While there are a large number of diseases that can be diagnosed *in utero,* unfortunately only a very small fraction can be treated then. Is its use moral?

> If prenatal diagnosis respects the life and integrity of the embryo and the human fetus and is directed toward its safeguarding or healing as an individual, then the answer is affirmative.[20]

Thus the only valid purpose of prenatal diagnosis is to identify a problem and to help individuals begin to deal with it. The parents must be informed, give their consent, and there can be no disproportionate risks. One may not request or advise prenatal diagnosis if the results may lead to an abortion. Similarly, there should be no directives or programs of the state or of medical organizations that link prenatal diagnosis and abortion. The fetus has a right to life and this cannot be compromised.

2. Research and Experimentation

Here the instruction distinguishes between these procedures *in vivo* and *in vitro*.

With respect to embryos and fetuses *in vivo,*

> If the embryos are living, whether viable or not, they must be respected just like any other human person; experimentation on embryos which is not directly therapeutic is illicit.[21]

Thus for the fetus in the uterus, research and therapy can be done if there is "a moral certainty of not causing harm to the life or integrity of the child and mother . . ."[22] and consent is given. In addition, no means, however noble or great, can justify the manipulation of an embryo or fetus.

With respect to research conducted *in vitro,* the instruction gives a clear prohibition: "It is immoral to produce human embryos destined to be exploited as disposable 'biological material.' "[23] Two moral issues are involved here. The first is the prohibition of reducing humans to means. The second is the voluntary exposure to death of embryos obtained *in vitro.* Such embryos, either specifically created for research or so-called spare embryos remaining after an IVF attempt, are "exposed to an absurd fate, with no possibility of their being offered safe means of survival which can be licitly pursued."[24]

Thus research on embryos or fetuses is very tightly regulated. The only justification for such research is the moral probability of a therapeutic benefit. All other interventions are prohibited.

3. *Heterologous Artificial Fertilization*

Every pregnancy must occur within heterosexual marriage and be the result of the conjugal act between the husband and wife. Thus,

> Heterologus artificial fertilization is contrary to the unity of marriage, to the dignity of the spouses, to the vocation proper to parents, and to the child's right to be conceived and brought into the world in marriage and from marriage.[25]

As noted previously, such a method of conception also violates the rights of the child, compromises his or her parental origins, and can interfere with the development of personal identity.[26] This position eliminates any use of donor semen whether for artificial insemination or for IVF.

This same reasoning applies, obviously, to the case of surrogate motherhood. Its practice violates several of the previously discussed moral values.

> Surrogate motherhood represents an objective failure to meet the obligation of maternal love, of conjugal fidelity and of responsible motherhood; it offends the dignity and the right of the child to be conceived, carried in the womb, brought into the world and brought up by his own parents; it sets up, to the detriment of families, a division between the physical, psychological and moral elements which constitute those families.[27]

Surrogacy, therefore, separates everything that the natural-law tradition would see as inherently joined and, consequently, violates a substantive moral norm.

4. Homologous Artificial Fertilization

One can evaluate this technique either *in vitro* or *in vivo*. The question is whether or not the husband's semen is to be used for artificial insemination or for IVF. The key to the moral analysis is

> 'the inseparable connection, willed by God and unable to be broken by man on his own initiative, between the two meanings of the conjugal act: the unitive meaning and the procreative meaning. Indeed, by its intimate structure the conjugal act, while most closely uniting husband and wife, capacitates them for the generation of new lives according to laws inscribed in the very being of man and of woman'.[28]

Any sexual act performed between the husband and wife

must preserve both the procreative possibility and the conjugal relation. Conversely, "procreation is deprived of its proper perfection when it is not desired as the fruit of the conjugal act, that is to say, of the specific act of the spouses' union."[29] Consequently,

> . . . the generation of a child must therefore be the fruit of that mutual giving which is realized in the conjugal act wherein the spouses cooperate as servants and not as masters in the work of the Creator, who is love.[30]

Artificial insemination with the husband's sperm is prohibited because of the separation of the unitive and procreative dimensions of the conjugal act and because the semen is typically obtained through masturbation, a further separation of these two normative aspects of married intercourse. IVF with the husband's semen is also prohibited.

> Such fertilization is neither in fact achieved nor positively willed as the expression and fruit of a specific act of the conjugal union. In homologous *'in vitro'* fertilization and embryo transfer, therefore, even if it is considered in the context of de facto existing sexual relations, the generation of the human person is objectively deprived of its proper perfection: namely, that of being the result and fruit of a conjugal act in which the spouses can become 'cooperators with God for giving life to a new person.'[31]

In addition, IVF establishes "the domination of technology over the origin and destiny of the human person."[32] As such it gives the "life and identity of the embryo into the power of doctors and biologists . . ."[33] Consequently, the dignity of parents and child is lost.

Finally, associated with IVF are two other practices that the instruction considers wrong. First is the practice either of allowing to die or of disposing of the fertilized eggs which were not chosen for implantation. This is essentially a procured abortion and, therefore, prohibited.[34] Second, the instruction also prohibits the freezing, or cryopreservation, of embryos. This practice, proposed by many as the solution to the first practice, is prohibited because it violates the respect due humans by

> exposing them to grave risks of death or harm to their physical integrity and depriving them, at least temporarily, of maternal shelter and gestation, thus placing them in a situation in which further offenses and manipulation are possible.[35]

Again the key moral principles are the dignity of the person—embryo, husband, and wife—and the inseparable union of the procreative and unitive dimension of the conjugal act.

5. *Permissible Means*

While the instruction does not identify specifically any particular means that could licitly be used, it does identify the moral principle by which to test a means to assist reproduction:

> If the technical means facilitates the conjugal act or helps it to reach its natural objectives, it can be morally acceptable. If, on the other hand, the procedure were to replace the conjugal act, it is morally illicit.[36]

Thus, as long as the means used respects the natural unity of the unitive and procreative dimensions of the conjugal act and does not suggest the manufacture of life, the technique is licit. For example, according to this norm, the previously noted procedure of LTOT would be licit because it simply involves the removal of an egg and replacing it in an appropriate place in the Fallopian tube so that it can be fertilized *in vivo*. Thus conception is only assisted; fertilization occurs in the customary way and preserves the natural unity of the conjugal act. Another procedure that has customarily been permitted is the cervical cap or spoon which places semen, collected after the conjugal act is completed, further in the vaginal tract to facilitate conception. Sperm could also be obtained, some have argued, from a perforated condom and then placed in the vaginal tract so conception could occur.

In any event, the critical moral test is whether the procedure 1) respects the natural unity of the procreative and unitive elements of the conjugal act; 2) assists in facilitating conception; 3) respects the dignity of all involved.

SUMMARY

The instruction is quite clear in its judgment on the reproductive technologies. The judgment is a rather clear and unambiguous "No." This analysis, though augmented by modern concepts of human dignity and moral rights, relies quite heavily on the traditional natural-law analysis of the nature of intercourse having an inseparable procreative and unitive dimension. There can, therefore, be absolutely no separation of any dimension of any aspect of reproduction. Consequently, the instruction prohibits IVF, ET, surrogate motherhood, cryopreservation of embryos, and most research on embryos and fetuses.

4.

A Comparative Analysis

This chapter will review American, Australian, and British guidelines to provide an overview of other perspectives on this topic and to establish the basis for a comparative evaluation of the Vatican "Instruction on Respect for Human Life in Its Origin and on the Dignity of Procreation."[1] These guidelines come from legislation, proposals for national policy, professional groups, or research centers. Of critical significance, for both ethical analysis and public-policy implementations, are the differences in anthropological assumptions between the instruction and these other documents. Some of these issues will be identified to help set a context for reading the documents and to indicate in general how they differ from the instruction.

In particular the American, British, and Australian legislative and professional documents self-consciously assume pluralistic audiences and attempt to identify some moral values or general moral principles on the basis of which public policy could be set. The value frequently appealed to in these three sets of documents is freedom of choice. This value is then associated with other socially approved values such as, for example, privacy, autonomy, and self-determination. This cluster reflects dominant cultural values that form the basis for social consensus which can then serve as the foundation for public policy.

The method frequently used for resolving social disputes concerning the implementation of these values is, however, consequentialism or pragmatism, based on assumptions about social consensus. This is how benefit/burden or cost/benefit calculations are made or value conflicts resolved. Frequently the values of freedom and privacy, as well as the assumed social consensus around certain issues, will be used to resolve a debate about a specific policy. This is a procedural solution, however, that may in fact not resolve the moral issues surrounding artificial reproduction.

For example, in the American Fertility Society's document, the phrase "human nature" is not used as a category of moral analysis even though it is explicitly identified as such in chapter five of the document. Such a normative reading of this phrase might have been avoided because it is easy to read various anthropologies into the phrase or because the phrase is identified with a particular tradition and its interpretation, i.e., the instruction. Yet, as just noted, some concept of human nature and framework is operative. The AFS document frequently highlights freedom and autonomy and particularly understands them as rights to be exercised by the individual. In addition, the document understands happiness as the achievement of immediate needs and goals. Finally, technology is seen as an appropriate means through which human freedom can achieve this understanding of happiness. The British policy suggested in the Warnock Report, although explicitly operating on the moral theory of sentiment, also makes normative claims about preembryonic life even though they are not substantively justified. And surrogacy is separated from IVF in the Australian guidelines on the basis of lack of consensus, but neither its formation nor its basis is reported.

Thus certain understandings of values or a particular model

of human nature are *implicitly* appealed to while *explicitly* no such content is evaluated. The documents considered below in particular downplay the concept of a physical "nature," reject some set of normative characteristics that frame human behavior, and do not assert any moral significance to personal relations based on or derived from physical relations. The comments on surrogacy in all three documents are somewhat of an exception to this latter point, but even in this case, all the guidelines are reluctant to interfere with happiness and choice. Again the category of choice and a sense of the person independent from his or her bodily dimension set the tone for the analysis. Dissatisfaction with this approach is noted in the AFS report in appendix A, written by Richard McCormick, S. J., who is also the author of the chapter on human nature. In this appendix, McCormick argues against various forms of third-party reproduction explicitly from a normative understanding of human nature as well as a consideration of the consequences of such practices. Thus in the AFS report we can see two understandings of human nature in conflict with each other but with no means provided by which to resolve the tension.

These documents, then, should be understood primarily as procedural guidelines designed either to identify social consensus or to use that consensus as the basis for resolving disputed points of public policy. Ironically, however, all the documents assume a certain view of "human nature" even though they, unlike the instruction, do not explicitly identify it.

AMERICAN REGULATIONS

Ethics Advisory Board of the Department of Health, Education and Welfare. 1979.[2]

The Ethics Advisory Board (EAB) was established on the recommendation of a previous presidential bioethical commission. Its purpose was to review certain bioethical questions of national importance. One of the first questions examined was that of IVF and embryo transfer.[3] In its conclusions, the EAB discussed three issues: 1) the ethical acceptability of such procedures; 2) a discussion of several areas of concern; and 3) their conclusions with respect to IVF and ET.

The EAB defined two senses of "ethical acceptability." The first sense is that of "clearly ethically right" and the second is "ethically defensible but still legitimately controverted."[4] The EAB used the second meaning in arguing that IVF and ET are ethically acceptable. By this the EAB intended to assert that there are significant ethical problems associated with IVF and ET, but that there were also substantive benefits stemming from the procedures.

Next, the EAB discussed four areas of concern. The first was the moral status of the embryo. Here the EAB concluded:

> The Board is in agreement that the human embryo is entitled to profound respect; but this respect does not necessarily encompass the full legal and moral rights attributed to persons.[5]

In addition, because of the high rate of embryo loss occurring in customary reproduction, the EAB concluded that some embryo loss in the attempts of an infertile couple to obtain children of their own was acceptable under certain conditions.

Concerns about safety of the mother and embryo were also raised. Because the procedures were quite new then, many questions had not been resolved and the HEW determined that "it has a legitimate interest in developing and disseminating information regarding safety and health so that fully informed choices about reproduction can be made."[6] While many of the concerns identified at that time have been resolved and the procedures shown to be relatively risk free,

nonetheless the concern of the EAB is well taken and continuous monitoring should occur.

The EAB then discussed the implications and applications
of these technologies. Issues raised included genetic manipulation, cloning, casual experimentation, the creation of genetic hybrids, and surrogate mothers. Although the EAB
recognized the potential for abuse, it concluded that "a broad
prohibition of research involving human *in vitro* fertilization
is neither wise nor justified."[7] The EAB saw legislation, regulation, and good judgment as more appropriate means of
curbing abuses. The EAB also noted that ". . . it is important
to guard against unwarranted governmental intrusion into
personal and marital privacy."[8]

Finally, the EAB considered whether or not the federal
government should support IVF and ET. While such funding
is objectionable to many because of their moral evaluation of
the embryo, nonetheless by funding such research, HEW
could help resolve many of the safety questions and ensure
that the research is carried on in an appropriate fashion. The
EAB, however, concluded

> that it should not advise the Department on the level of
> Federal support, if any, of such research; but it concluded
> that Federal support, if decided upon after due consid-
> eration of all that is at issue, would be acceptable from
> an ethical standpoint.[9]

At a later date, a research protocol involving human embryos and IVF was submitted to HEW and referred to the
EAB. The decision was not to fund such research, and this
still remains the policy at HHS.

Given this review, the EAB then drew several conclusions.

> (1) The Department should consider support of more an-
> imal research in order to assess the risks to both mother

and offspring associated with the procedures; (2) the conduct of research involving human *in vitro* fertilization designed to establish the safety and effectiveness of the procedure is ethically acceptable under certain conditions; (3) Departmental support of such research would be acceptable from an ethical standpoint, although the Board did not address the question of the level of funding, if any, which such research might be given; (4) the Department should take the initiative in collecting, analyzing and disseminating data from both research and clinical practice involving *in vitro* fertilization throughout the world; and (5) model or uniform laws should be developed to define the rights and responsibilities of all parties involved in such activities.[10]

The EAB then specified the conditions under which HEW could support such research. These are:

A. If the research involves human *in vitro* fertilization without embryo transfer, the following conditions are satisfied.

1. The research complies with all appropriate provisions of the regulations governing research with human subjects (45 CFR 46);

2. The research is designed primarily: (A) To establish the safety and efficacy of embryo transfer and (B) to obtain important scientific information toward that end not reasonably attainable by other means;

3. Human gametes used in such research will be obtained exclusively from persons who have been informed of the nature and purpose of the research in which such materials will be used and have specifically consented to such use;

4. No embryos will be sustained *in vitro* beyond the stage normally associated with the completion of implantation (14 days after fertilization) and;

5. All interested parties and the general public will be advised if evidence begins to show that the procedure

entails risks of abnormal offspring higher than those associated with natural human reproduction.

B. In addition, if the research involves embryo transfer
following human *in vitro* fertilization, embryo transfer
will be attempted only with gametes obtained from law-
fully married couples.[11]

These are the guidelines currently in place with respect to
federal funding of IVF and ET. In addition, since no research
has been supported, there is a de facto moratorium on public
research in these areas. Existing research and/or clinical practice are funded privately.

American College of Obstetricians and Gynecologists

In 1983, the American College of Obstetricians and Gynecologists (ACOG) issued a set of professional guidelines concerning surrogate motherhood.[12] While addressing only one
facet of the broader question of artificial reproduction, the
policy statement presents another model of an ethical analysis
of a particular problem.

The concerns addressed in the document include: the de-
personalization of reproduction, the stress on the infertile
couple, the potential for eugenic manipulation, the potential
impact of the technologies on the children, and the need for
anonymity. Specific concerns were also raised about the regulation of a surrogate pregnancy, the effects of the separation
of the infant from the surrogate, the question of who is to
receive medical information about the pregnancy and who is
to be the decision maker, questions of abortion, and the question of what to do with the infant if the rearing parents do
not want it. In addition, ACOG raises three specific problems
in the use of surrogacy for convenience: 1) an increase in de-
personalization; 2) a surrogate's bearing a risk that could be
borne by the couple; and 3) questions about the dedication

to parenthood in the couple contracting for a baby to be born of a surrogate.

With these concerns in mind, ACOG made recommendations regarding surrogate arrangements and the care of pregnant surrogates.

I. Initiation of Surrogate Arrangements.

A. When approached by a patient interested in surrogate motherhood, the physician should, as in all other aspects of medical care, be certain there is a full discussion of ethical and medical risks, benefits and alternatives.

B. A physician may justifiably decline to participate in surrogate motherhood arrangements.

C. If a physician decides to become involved in a surrogate-motherhood arrangement, he or she should follow these guidelines:

1. The physician should be assured that appropriate procedures are utilized to screen the contracting couple and the surrogate. Such screening may include appropriate fertility studies and genetic screening.

2. The physician should receive only the usual compensation for obstetric and gynecologic services. Referral fees and other arrangements for financial gain beyond the usual fees for medical services are inappropriate.

3. The physician should not participate in a surrogate program where the financial arrangements are likely to exploit any of the parties.

II. Care of Pregnant Surrogates.

A. When a woman seeks medical care for an established pregnancy, regardless of the method of conception, she should be cared for as any other obstetric patient or referred to a qualified physician who will provide that care.

B. The surrogate mother should be considered the source of consent with respect to clinical intervention and management of the pregnancy. Confidentiality between the physician and patient should be maintained. If other parties, such as the adoptive parents, are to play a role

in decision making, the parameters should be clearly de-
lineated, with the agreement of the patient.[13]

The essential constraints on the physician have to do with
his or her individual acceptance of the procedure and then,
if he or she agrees to be the physician, to be attentive to the
rights of all parties. In addition, the physician is not to increase
his or her standard fees because of the surrogacy situation.

American Fertility Society

"Ethical Considerations of the New Reproductive Technologies" was issued by the Ethics Committee of the American Fertility Society (AFS) in September 1986.[14] The Committee was formed in 1984, held eight formal sessions, and
then issued its statement in 1986. This section will identify
the ethical principles relevant to the issues and will summarize
the Committee's conclusions of various procedures.[15]

ETHICAL PRINCIPLES
The basic ethical principle used to evaluate artificial reproduction is *"the human person integrally and adequately considered."*[16] This approach focuses on human well-being: bodily,
intellectually, spiritually, and socially. The criterion situates
itself in the intersection of the major social institutions: family,
economy, politics, and religion. Actions that undermine the
person in these essential dimensions are wrong; actions that
promote and support the person are right.

There are some features of this criterion that are important.
First, the criterion requires "an inductive approach based on
experience and reflection."[17] This suggests that one needs to
consider the comprehensive impact of acts on persons to develop a full moral understanding of the action. Second, some
acts will remain ambiguous because they "involve both beneficial and detrimental aspects, because their impact on persons
is unknown, or because they are variously evaluated."[18] This
reality calls for attitudes of openness, caution, and a willing-

ness to revise one's original opinion. Finally, the criterion takes into account the fact that the "person is both individual and social."[19] Thus one cannot look exclusively at the individual for a full moral evaluation of the act, but one also needs to take into account, as far as possible, the social consequences.

A second ethical principle, derived from constitutional law, is the right to procreate. Such a right, while not yet having full constitutional sanctioning, appears to be a fundamental human right. Such a right would "protect individual procreative choice unless there is a compelling need for state intervention."[20] Such a right, typically applied to married heterosexual couples, would protect individuals who sought to reproduce by other means. Such a right is a liberty right and would not mandate state action to assist couples who are seeking to reproduce by whatever means.[21]

While noting that there are virtually no constraints on one's legal liberty right to reproduce, the report notes that there may be moral limitations.[22] Six are noted: the transmission of disease to offspring, unwillingness to provide proper prenatal care, inability to rear children, psychological harm to offspring, overpopulation, and nonmarriage. The dominant concern here is harm, not only to the child but also to society. Thus the report concluded that "couples have a liberty right to reproduce, limited by ethical constraints."[23]

A third ethical concern is the moral status of the preembryo.[24] Three views are noted: 1) the according of full human status and rights to the preembryo; 2) considering the preembryo no different than any other human tissue; 3) the middle view of assigning the preembryo greater respect than afforded other human tissue, but not granting it full personal status.[25]

The Committee noted that there is wide consensus that the preembryo has a special moral status, but is not equivalent to a person.

> Therefore, we find a widespread consensus that the preembryo is not a person but is to be treated with special

respect because it is a genetically unique, living human entity that might become a person.[26]

A fourth ethical issue discusses a new development: patents in reproductive medicine. Patenting a procedure or a technology in medicine raises several problems. For example, how can one precisely identify whether a process is a genuinely new procedure or a variation on an existing procedure? Also, patenting a procedure would make the training of new physicians very difficult. One would need to receive permission or pay a royalty each time the procedure was used. This might then create an incentive to use an unpatented procedure, even though the patented procedure is more appropriate. In addition, enforcement would prove difficult. Finally, the patient would suffer because of increased costs and violations of privacy in enduring enforcement. Thus the Committee recommends that patents not be sought on diagnostic or therapeutic procedures.[27]

POLICY RECOMMENDATIONS

The Committee identified many instances of artificial reproduction, described and discussed them, and then made a specific recommendation. For the sake of simplicity, I will identify the procedure and state as succinctly as possible the conclusion(s) drawn.

1. In Vitro *Fertilization.* Since the Committee found no persuasive evidence of harm to the child or couple from IVF, since IVF can be seen as an extension of sexual intimacy, and because possible abuses of a technology do not invalidate appropriate use, the "Committee unamiously finds that basic IVF is ethically acceptable."[28]

2. *Artificial insemination.* Three instances of AI are considered: the husband, a donor, and donor with IVF.

With respect to artificial insemination with the husband's sperm (AIH), for demonstrated medical indications such as impotence, vaginal dysfunction, or erectile dysfunction consequent to various drug therapies, AIH is acceptable. With respect to uncertain indications such as cervical mucus abnormalities, poor sperm motility, problems of spermatogenesis, AIH should be considered as a clinical trial that should be followed carefully.

Although the first use of artificial insemination with a donor (AID) can be documented as early as the nineteenth century, widespread use did not come until later. The main issues with AID are the use of third-party gametes with the potential of harm to the child, the husband, and the introduction of a risk of the transmission of genetic disease unless appropriate screening is done. Since AID provides a child with a genetic link to the wife and because adoption is a difficult process, the Committee "finds the use of AID ethically acceptable."[29] The Committee additionally recommends that the couple be given adequate information, that a permanent record be designed to preserve confidentiality and anonymity, and that the same donor not be used for more than ten offspring.

The Committee notes two reasons for the use of donor sperm in IVF: 1) the woman has an "infertility factor that necessitates IVF technology and her partner is a subfertile or infertile man . . .";[30] 2) donor sperm may be used as a backup if the "man's fertilizing potential is unknown or suspect . . ."[31]. The Committee accepts the use of donor sperm in IVF as ethically acceptable, but views it as a backup in the situations described above.

3. *Donor eggs in IVF.* The use of donor eggs arises when a woman is unable to provide her own eggs or when her eggs have a genetic defect. Many of the concerns of this situation are similar to those associated with AID. In addition, there are unresolved legal problems with respect to the determination of motherhood when a donor egg is used. Also, a woman undergoes several physical risks to have her eggs obtained.

The Committee found the use of donor eggs acceptable under certain conditions. These include: no compensation for the donor, the preservation of anonymity, taking extreme care in obtaining eggs from a woman undergoing laparoscopy only for the purpose of being an egg donor, and screening the eggs for genetic diseases.[32]

4. *Preembryos from IVF for donation.* The conditions in which this might be called for are rare: the female has indications for a donor egg and the male has indications for donor sperm. While the consequences of such a practice are unknown, the Committee notes that such preembryo donation more closely resembles traditional pregnancies in that the mother bears the pregnancy and then nurtures the child.

Thus the Committee finds this practice ethically acceptable with the provisos that there be no compensation, anonymity be maintained, and that screening for genetic diseases be done.[33]

5. *Uterine lavage for preembryo transfer.* In this procedure, a preembryo, formed through artificial insemination by the husband or a donor, is lavaged from the donor and transferred to the infertile woman so she can carry the pregnancy. Thus the procedure permits women with no eggs to carry a pregnancy and give birth.

Because of unclarity about the risk/benefit ratio of this procedure, the Committee recommends that it ". . . should be regarded as a clinical experiment and should require suitable review and oversight."[34] General application of the procedure is considered premature.

6. *Cryopreservation.* The Committee considers three specific cases of cryopreservation: sperm, egg, and preembryo.

The freezing of sperm has been done since 1953, and the success of the process has given rise to the international development of sperm banks. Although the practice is not without some controversary, the Committee found that the cryopreservation of sperm is ethically and medically acceptable.[35]

Attempts to freeze the egg have not met with success. This is due to the relatively large mass of cytoplasm that is usually harmed when frozen. Thus the Committee recommendation here focuses on the development of procedures to ensure the safe freezing of the egg. When preliminary research on this has been completed, then the "fertilization and/or transfer of cryopreserved eggs should be considered as a clinical experiment."[36]

The cryopreservation of embryos is controversial. While the procedure is somewhat successful—about 50 to 60 percent of human preembryos are viable after freezing and thawing[37]—society has yet to achieve any consensus of the issue. Cryopreservation resolves two problems: it prevents the destruction of surplus fertilized eggs, and it allows fertilized eggs to be saved for later use if the first IVF attempt fails. In making its recommendation, the Committee acknowledged the difficulty of balancing the medical justification and utility of frozen preembryos and the difficulty of rendering an ethical judgment on the procedure.

> The Committee therefore believes that research using cryopreservation techniques should be pursued, with careful oversight, in those centers that perform this type of research. It appears at present that a general clinical application of freezing human preembryos is inappropriate. The uses of human preembryo material for cryopreservation therefore should be viewed as a clinical experiment until such time as the success rate and preembryo risks are clearly defined.[38]

7. *Surrogacy.* In this report, the Committee discussed separately the surrogate gestational mother—the woman who provides the gestational component only—and the surrogate

mother—the woman who provides both the genetic and gestational component.

The primary indication for a surrogate gestational mother (SGM) is the lack of the gestational component for reproduction. Thus a woman may have no uterus or may be put at high risk were she to become pregnant. In this case, the woman's egg could be fertilized with her husband's sperm and then transferred to the SGM for the duration of the pregnancy.

Several reservations are considered. The SGM is put at risk without receiving compensating benefits; the SGM may be coerced into the situation and she may suffer psychological harm. The couple is also at risk of harm if the SGM will not surrender the baby, if the fetus is harmed by the SGM's activities, and the couple's relation to each other and to the child could be harmed should the SGM want continual involvement. Nonetheless, the SGM may be the last hope for a couple to have a child with a genetic link to them; the child is given the opportunity to exist; and it provides an opportunity for the SGM to practice altruism or to benefit themselves psychologically.[39]

After noting that SGM can present risks to all participants, that there are concerns about the payment of SGMs, and that the lack of laws in the area ensures little protection for the participants, the Committee recommends against SGM "for a nonmedical reason, such as the convenience of the genetic mother . . ."[40] because nonmedical reasons are inadequate to justify the risks of pregnancy and delivery. Room is left open in reproductive medicine, however, for SGM as a clinical experiment. If done in this fashion, several areas of research are identified: the psychological effects on the SGM, the couple, and the child; the possibility of bonding between the SGM and the fetus; the appropriate screening of the SGM and the couple; the likelihood that the SGM will care for herself properly during pregnancy; whether having the SGM and the couple meet or not makes any difference; the effects of being a SGM on her own family, if any; the effects of disclosing or not disclosing the use of a SGM or her identity to the child; and other issues that may become apparent during the procedure.[41]

Since being a surrogate mother (SM) requires only artificial insemination, the practice has frequently developed "in an entrepreneurial setting, generally apart from medical institutions."[42] The three indications for the use of an SM are the inability of a woman to provide either the genetic or gestational component of childbearing or either component separately. The reservations are similar to those raised with the SGM, in addition to potential complications derived from the child's genetic link to the SM. This also raises questions about privacy, the ethics of donor involvement, and the potential impact on the couple's marriage. Nonetheless, the practice of SM may be the husband's only opportunity to have a child with a genetic link to himself. That desire must be weighted against a variety of concerns: the risks to all the participants; the commercialization of the practice, including the use of brokers to facilitate the procedure; and the lack of laws to protect any of the participants. Thus the Committee recommends against the use of SMs for a nonmedical reason such as the convenience of the rearing mother. The risks of pregnancy and delivery are not outweighed by such a reason. Two medical reasons justify the use of an SM: ". . . the only medical solution to infertility in a couple of whom the woman has no uterus and who does not produce eggs or does not want to risk passing on a genetic defect that she carries."[43] If surrogacy is pursued in this fashion, it should be as a clinical experiment to generate data to help resolve the assessment of the possible risks and benefits of the procedure. The Committee recommends that the same research issues identified above for the SGM be used to study the surrogate mother. In addition, the Committee recommends that professionals accept only their typical fees, accept no finder's fees, and expresses the preference that surrogates not be compensated other than for medical and other similar expenses.[44]

8. *Quality assurance.* Because of the impacts of the reproductive technologies on individual and society as well as the profound ethical issues that they raise, the issue of quality assurance is most important. Thus it is extremely significant that the report discusses issues such as training, the standardization of the operations of the clinic, the importance of follow-up studies, record-keeping, the professional disclosure of statistics, and appropriate disclosure of relevant information to patients.[45] Such insistence on professional standards and the establishment of guidelines only serve to enhance the quality of care of all the participants in the reproductive technologies.

BRITISH GUIDELINES

Medical Research Council

A 1982 review of developments in artificial reproduction led to the British Medical Research Council's (MRC) statement supporting various forms of research on human pre-embryos. After determining that specific consent needed to be obtained for research purposes and that appropriate animal work should proceed research on humans, the MRC said:

> (i) Scientifically sound research involving experiments on the processes and products of *in vitro* fertilisation between human gametes is ethically acceptable and should be allowed to proceed on condition both that there is no intent to transfer to the uterus any embryo resulting from or used in such experiments and also that the aim of the

problems such as contraception or the differential diagnosis and treatment of infertility and inherited diseases.

(vi) Studies on interspecies fertilisation are valuable in
providing information on the penetration capacity and
chromosome complement of sperm from subfertile males,
and should be supported. The fertilised ova should not
be allowed to develop beyond the early cleavage stage.[46]

These guidelines very clearly and strongly supported the
use of preembryos in research in a wide variety of contexts.

British Medical Association

Also in 1982, the British Medical Association (BMA) issued
the "Interim Report of Human In Vitro Fertilisation and Embryo Replacement and Transfer." This examined the clinical
application of IVF as opposed to the research dimension considered by the MRC. After reviewing the technology, the
success rates, and its use, the BMA first recommended that
IVF be restricted to only a few centers that have the necessary
expertise. This would also facilitate keeping the records and
establishing the studies that BMA recommended be carried
out.

BMA made three specific recommendations regarding IVF
and surrogacy:

> (8) It is ethically acceptable to undertake *in vitro* fer-
> tilisation using the sperm and ova of the couple concerned
> with subsequent replacement in the uterus of the woman
> of the couple.
> (9) Given informed consent by all parties concerned,
> the use of donated sperm for *in vitro* fertilisation of the
> ovum of the female partner with embryo replacement in
> her uterus or the use of a donated ovum for *in vitro* fer-
> tilisation by the male partner's sperm with embryo trans-
> fer to the female partner is not unethical. In the rare case

in which neither party can produce viable gametes (sperm or ova), the use of donated sperm and donated ova for *in vitro* fertilisation and transfer to the female member of the couple may be ethically acceptable.

(13) The working group has yet to be satisfied that to undertake *in vitro* fertilisation with the sperm and ova of a couple and to transfer the embryo to the uterus of another woman who might carry the embryo to term on behalf of the couple will ever be acceptable. (The term "surrogate motherhood" has been applied to this situation and is distinct from the situation described in paragraph 9).[47]

BMA also accepted embryo storage by freezing, but stated that such storage should not last beyond twelve months, after which the couple's wishes for storage should be respected insofar as possible. In addition, IVF should not be used to transfer to a uterus a preembryo on which genetic manipulation had been done.

The Warnock Report

A committee was again formed in 1984 to consider these issues because of continuing technical accomplishments and applications. The resulting Warnock Report came up with sixty-four recommendations related to all aspects of artificial reproduction, research, IVF, surrogacy, and recommended laws.

ETHICAL PRINCIPLES

Perhaps because the Committee was headed by Dame Mary Warnock, an Oxford philosopher, now Mistress of Girton College, Cambridge, the ethical principles used in the evaluation are clearly articulated. In her introduction to the report, as well as in the body of the report itself, Warnock discusses the basic ethical method. She begins by recognizing that while it may be necessary to argue for some issues on a utilitarian basis, this theory cannot, by itself, resolve some critical questions, e.g., *"how to regard embryos."*[48] Also, blind obedience to rules in and of itself cannot resolve such issues. Therefore moral sentiment was invoked in order to sort out feelings and to attempt to justify them. Thus utilitarian arguments were not totally satisfactory and people's moral sentiments differ. "Therefore moral conflict may be unavoidable."[49]

After considering various positions on the moral status of the human embryo and examining what protection it has in law, the report concluded, although with dissent, that the human embryo in the UK is not accorded the same status as a living child or an adult. Nonetheless,

> we were agreed that the embryo of the human species ought to have a special status and that no one should undertake research on human embryos the purposes of which could be achieved by the use of other animals or in some other way. The status of the embryo is a matter of fundamental principle which should be enshrined in legislation.[50]

This protection is expressed through not allowing the embryo's maintenance outside the uterus for more than fourteen days *in vitro*. In addition, research on human embryos should be conducted only under the auspices of a licensing agency and any unauthorized use *in vitro* would be a criminal offense.[51]

POLICY RECOMMENDATIONS

Three specific areas are commented on in the report: AID and AIH, IVF, and surrogate motherhood.

The use of artificial insemination either by husband or donor is accepted by the report. The only restrictions come with

AID and these have to do with removing it from its current legal vacuum. Thus the report recommends a licensing agency, assurances of the consent of all parties, the legitimization of the child, registering the husband of the couple as the father, limiting to ten the number of children to be fathered by a donor, and making reimbursement only for fees.[52]

The report accepts IVF as an accepted treatment for infertility. It recommends, however, that it be subject to licensing as with AID and that it be available within the National Health Service. Egg donation, subject to the same regulation as AID and AIH, should also be accepted as treatment for infertility. Similarly, embryo donation with donor sperm and egg and IVF ought also to be accepted, subject to the previously mentioned licensing and controls. Because of risks to the egg donor, the Committee recommended against the use of embryo donation by lavage.[53]

Surrogate motherhood presented several concerns to the Committee. Among these were the use of surrogacy for the convenience of the rearing mother, the danger of potentially exploiting the surrogate, the treating of people as means, and the commercialization of surrogacy.

> We recommend that legislation be introduced to render criminal the creation or the operation in the United Kingdom of agencies whose purposes include the recruitment of women for surrogate pregnancies or making arrangements for individuals or couples who wish to utilize the services of a carrying mother; such legislation should be wide enough to include both profit and non-profit making organisations. We further recommend that the legislation be sufficiently wide to render criminally liable the actions of professionals and others who knowingly assist in the establishment of a surrogate pregnancy.[54]

This recommendation would not make private parties to

surrogate arrangements liable to prosecution, but would make all surrogacy arrangements legally unenforcable. Thus, while the children born of such arrangements would not be subject to the "taint of criminality,"[55] neither would such arrangements be encouraged.

With respect to cryopreservation, the Committee recommended the continued use of frozen sperm for use in AI, recommended against the use of frozen eggs until research shows a decrease in risks, and stated that the "clinical use of frozen embryos may continue to be developed under review by the licensing board."[56] Also, maximum storage time for embryos should be ten years; the right to disposal resides with the couple who stored the embryo; and most importantly, the Committee argued that "legislation be enacted to ensure there is no right of ownership in a human embryo."[57]

The Warnock Report essentially sanctions the continuation of the new technologies. In part this is because many of these have strong public support and in part because the procedures present no substantive risk of harm. The line is drawn, however, at the commercialization of surrogate motherhood. The Committee saw this procedure as simply having too many problems and little social support.

The Warnock Report also favored establishing a licensing board to monitor, study, and regulate the implementation of many of these technologies. In this way the technologies can be controlled without either stopping significant developments or putting so many obstacles in the way of scientists and/or clinicians that progress is discouraged.

Finally, the Committee made a clear determination about the moral status of the human embryo. It recognized that it has a unique value because of its potential, but the Committee stopped short of equating the value of the preembryo with an individual existing outside of the uterus. Nonetheless, this valuing of the preembryo is the foundation for many of the moral restraints in the report.

AUSTRALIAN GUIDELINES

Australia is one of the leaders in the development and application of the birth technologies. Consequently, several sets of guidelines have been developed there. We will conclude our review of regulations by considering several of these.

National Health and Medical Research Council, 1982.

While recognizing that IVF is a justifiable means of treating infertility, the Council also recognized that much research needs to be done. Therefore every center using these procedures should have an ethics committee to review all attempts to secure pregnancies in this fashion. Also a registry should be established to monitor the outcomes.

IVF is a recognized procedure and normally will occur within an established family and with the egg and sperm of the partners.[58] Should the ovum be unsuitable, however, the woman could receive a donated egg if the treatment occurs within an accepted familial relation, the couple accept the obligations of parenthood, all parties consent to the procedure, and the relation is not commercialized.[59] The Council said:

> A woman could produce a child for an infertile couple from ova and sperm derived from that couple. Because of current inability to determine or define motherhood in this context, this situation is not yet capable of ethical resolution.[60]

The Council also permits research on the preembryo up until the time when implantation would normally occur, and cryopreservation of preembryos for a period of about ten years but not beyond the "time of conventional reproductive need or competence of the female donor."[61] Finally, cloning experiments are prohibited, and those who conscientiously object to any of the procedures should neither be obligated to participate in them nor be put at an employment disadvantage because of their objections.

Victorian Government Committee: IVF, 1982.

This Committee focused its attention on IVF as practiced in Victoria, Australia, and based its recommendation on what it saw as acceptable there. While other issues needed to be considered, the report focused on the most common context of IVF in Victoria.

Consequently, the recommendation included setting up centers where IVF would be performed after other efforts to resolve infertility failed. Only married couples were to be admitted into the program, and "the gametes are obtained from husband and wife and the embryos are transferred into the uterus of the wife. . . ."[62]

Victorian Government Committee: Donor Gametes, 1983.

This report focused specifically on the role of donor gametes in IVF, thus taking the topic one step beyond the previous report.

After receiving appropriate information and giving consent, donor sperm and ova are ethically acceptable in IVF. Also a registry should be established containing information about the donors and the outcomes of pregnancies established through donors. And "It should be unlawful for donor embryos to be used except in the case of couples whose infertility cannot be overcome by other means, or where the couple may transmit undesirable hereditary disorders."[63] Finally, the gametes of donors should not be used to create a donor embryo, unless specific written consent is given for this use.

Victorian Government Committee:
Social, Ethical, and Legal Issues, 1984.

This set of guidelines focuses on the cryopreservation of preembryos and in general approves the practice. With this, the report recommends research on techniques for freezing and storage of the preembryo. Hospitals may not, however, dispose of these preembryos as they see fit. In addition, the preembryo can be frozen only if the couple from whom the gametes came agreed to the procedure. Also, "the couple whose gametes are used may not sell or casually dispose of the embryo."[64]

The couple from whom the gametes came are essentially responsible for the disposition of the frozen preembryo. If they consent, for example, the preembryo may be donated. Their decision for long-term storage is to be reviewed after five years, and they must determine the fate of the preembryos in the event of accident, death, or dissolution.

Two other recommendations deal with surrogacy:

> 6.17 A hospital licensed to conduct an IVF program shall not be permitted to make any commercial surrogacy arrangements as part of that programme.
> 6.18 Surrogacy arrangements shall in no circumstances be made at present as part of an IVF programme.[65]

Thus while IVF, as well as the use of donor ova and sperm, have a place in the resolution of childlessness, surrogacy is at present barred from being a part of the programs run in established centers in Victoria.

The recommendations in these three reports have been incorporated in the Infertility (Medical Procedures) Act of 1984.[66] In essence, IVF may be performed only at approved hospitals, for married couples for whom other infertility treatments have been unsuccessful and who have had counseling. Records are to be maintained with respect to pregnancies and donors.

This act also upholds the ban on commercial surrogacy. Any such contracts are void and unenforceable. "The act of

1984 prohibits both advertisements soliciting or offering surrogate-mother services and the giving or the receiving of any payments or rewards for such services."[67] This act does not cover altruistic or volunteer surrogacy.

While allowing embryo experimentation, the act also prohibits cloning, cross-species fertilization, the use of gametes produced by a child, IVF or AI with the sperm from more than one man, and the production of preembryos exclusively for the purpose of experimentation.

Finally, the act provides for the establishment of an eight-member Standing Review and Advisory Committee. The members are to be interdisciplinary and appointed by the minister of health. It is advisory with respect to infertility and its resolution and has "a special responsibility to consider requests for approval of experimental procedures involving embryos. . . ."[68]

Thus the Victoria community has responded to the new birth technologies with a set of recommendations from various committees, a set of laws, and an oversight panel to monitor, review, and update the current situation.

A COMPARATIVE ANALYSIS

Method

The sharpest difference between the various sets of regulations is present in the Vatican instruction and the guidelines of the American Fertility Society (AFS). Both have an explicit value perspective from which they begin their analysis, but this point of departure as well as the conclusions drawn differ considerably. The instruction appeals to two principles—human dignity and the inseparable procreative and unitive dimensions of intercourse—while the AFS appeals to human dignity integrally and adequately considered.

In the instruction, the second principle is a specification of the first principle with regard to human sexuality, and determines what "dignity" is to mean in the concrete. Our judgment is that the physical integrity of the act of intercourse is the ultimate criterion for judging the birth technologies. First, this principle has been the traditional principle appealed to in major teachings on marriage and reproduction, such as *Casti Connubii* and *Humanae Vitae*. Second, in the text, the argument is that respecting this natural unity is a way of showing respect for human dignity. Third, in the critical discussions of the morality of specific acts such as AID or AIH or IVF, the criterion appealed to is integrity of marital intercourse. Finally, the moral judgments are consequent to an evaluation of each and every separate act of intercourse. That is, the morality of the use of a birth technology cannot be evaluated from its perspective within the totality of the marriage, but must be judged on the basis of each individual act of intercourse. Consequently the absolute ban on any of the birth technologies follows very logically from this major premise of the inseparability of the unitive and procreative dimensions of intercourse.

The AFS, on the other hand, with its criterion of the dignity of the human integrally and adequately considered is more open to various birth technologies. For example, the guidelines typically look for evidence that a particular application will harm human dignity. The evidence is to be both empirical and principled. Thus, with respect to the practice of surrogacy, the AFS presents principled arguments why it should be prohibited, as well as suggesting empirical reasons that lead to its prohibition. Because the AFS looks at the person as a dynamic entity, its moral evaluation also considers the totality of the life situation of the individuals using the technologies. The AFS typically considers the technologies to be used within the context of a marriage and sees their use as a morally legitimate means of achieving the procreative dimension of marriage. The AFS is, however, willing to allow much more freedom of choice to the partners as they fulfill their legitimate desires to have children of their own. For instance, it would allow the involvement of ovum, sperm, and embryo donors from outside the marriage. Thus, for the AFS, protecting freedom of choice is a means of showing respect for the person. But freedom may be limited in view of social considerations, with such considerations defined primarily in terms of risk to the future freedom or social welfare of others who did not consent to the original practice of a technology. Finally, one must also evaluate the birth technologies from their social implications. This also gives a broader base from which judge their morality.

Thus the critical difference between the instruction and the AFS is methodological. The instruction identifies the integrity of the procreative and unitive dimensions of intercourse as the key, while the AFS focuses on the freedom of persons to choose to procreate by any means that do not violate the autonomy and consent of others. Although the AFS report employs a traditionally Catholic category ("nature"), supplied by Richard McCormick from *Gaudium et Spes,* the category is given substance primarily in terms of self-determination, while the instruction relies primarily on physical integrity. It is no surprise, therefore, that the instruction prohibits all birth technologies—since in fact they are premised on a separation of the act of intercourse into discrete elements—while the AFS approves most of them, without seeing physical nature as an appropriate limit on what can be included under "the nature of the person integrally and adequately considered." This divergence makes it clear that basic moral terms such as "dignity" and "nature" must be filled out carefully and critically, with attention to presupposed values.

The Warnock Report also utilized explicit moral methods. Essentially these were a combination of moral sentiment and utilitarianism. The report recognized that risk/benefit analysis in and of itself was inadequate to resolve comprehensively the problems associated with the birth technologies. One has to appeal to some standards in making these calculations and they do not come from utilitarianism. Therefore, one must appeal to moral sentiment, the dominant moral feelings of a people, as the standard by which to measure and judge one's calculations. Such a moral standard recognizes diversity of conclusions but also affirms a set of parameters within which those conclusions can be drawn.

Thus the report is liberal on the general uses of the birth technologies within marriage but sets this within a context of respect for the embryo and social regulation. While, generally speaking, individuals are free to choose, they can choose only within a certain framework. The report envisions, for example, that society should not sanction or protect surrogacy arrangements. Surrogacy is perceived as inherently problematic, especially because of its commercial dimensions and because of the possibility of professionals becoming brokers of infants. Thus, while the report does not prohibit individuals from making voluntary arrangements, it argues that society should have no part of supporting these choices.

The Australian regulations are less explicit in their methodology. The primary ethical value explicitly identified is the right of professionals to refuse to participate in such procedures. In addition, there is the assertion that the preembryo is to be protected, for example by a prohibition of research after the normal time of implantation; but there is no full account of why this should be so. Also surrogacy is not allowed to be linked to IVF programs, typically on the ground that there is no ethical resolution of it. How this judgment was reached or how one would know when there was an adequate resolution is left unstated. By inference, one can suggest that the essential value appealed to is freedom of choice. The morality of the birth technologies seems to be, in the Australian documents, that because the technologies are accepted medical treatments for infertility, their use is up to the individual. Thus, as long as consent is adequately obtained, the moral issues are resolved.

Areas of Conflict

The major area of conflict between the various regulations is over the evaluation of the moral status of the embryo. The instruction, for example, accords absolute value to the embryo in that this entity is accorded all rights of adult humans from the moment of conception. The instruction's position is that conception is the definitive beginning point of personal existence and from that time forward the preembryo must be accorded full human rights. This position leads to an absolute ban on research, the freezing of the preembryo, as well as any IVF or ET. Procedures that may be therapeutic but are experimental must also be shown to confer a likelihood of benefits before they can be used.

The other documents reviewed affirm a special status to the preembryo because it is of human origin and because it will develop into a human person. Nonetheless a critical dividing line is the stage of implantation, after which the individuality of the preembryo is fixed. During this time, the other documents allow research to occur, permit therapies to be applied, and allow IVF and ET. Freezing of the preembryo is also permitted. Thus, while the human preembryo is to be treated with care and shown respect, such care and respect are not absolute. Therefore, within the limit of the establishment of individuality, certain procedures are possible.

The other major value difference between the instruction and the other documents is the role of freedom of choice. The regulations reviewed assume that a critical value dimension is that of freedom. Individuals exercise choices with respect to reproductive rights; they exercise choices about when and under what circumstances they will reproduce; and they exercise control over the disposition of their gametes and preembryos that may be formed from them. Thus freedom of choice about means and ends is both a dominant value and a major cultural assumption running through the various documents.

The instruction, however, qualifies significantly one's choices by the nature of the conjugal act and the absolute value of the preembryo. Thus one can choose, but only within a narrowly prescribed range of moral options. The preembryo cannot, therefore, be reduced to a means to an end nor can the inherent unity of the conjugal act be disrupted, even for the best of reasons. Thus, while the instruction values freedom, it values the preembryo and the integrity of the conjugal act more. These two values stand as the test for the morality of one's choices.

A third area of dispute between the instruction and the other documents is the extent to which the state should regulate the various birth technologies. The Warnock Report is the closest to the instruction in wanting a licensing agency to regulate and monitor the use of the technologies. The purpose of the agency is primarily to ensure that standards are maintained, to determine whether follow-up studies need to be done, and to establish a moral framework acceptable to society as the basis on which both the status quo and future developments can be evaluated.

The instruction goes further and states that civil legislation is bound by the moral law and must conform to it. Therefore civil legislation is to be guided and based on the values proposed in the instruction. Thus the expectation coming from the Vatican is that restrictive legislation will be enacted that will protect the preembryo by prohibiting the use of various forms of the birth technologies.

The other documents recognize a need for some control, but since they identify the procedures as medical and under professional supervision and control, they do not see as much need for social supervision or control. Nonetheless, the

American Fertility Society, for example, recognizes that surrogacy is a controversial issue and that research needs to be done and that professionals ought to be careful about entering into or being part of surrogacy arrangements. It does not recommend, however, that the practice be prohibited or unduly restricted.

Social Evaluation of Technology

In addition to the value or methodological issues, perhaps the point of sharpest disagreement between the instruction and the other documents is on the point of the social evaluation of technology. In general, the various documents acknowledge that these new technologies will have profound influences on marriage and reproduction and have far-reaching social consequences. The dominant bases for interpreting the technologies, however, blunt any social critique. First, the technologies are typically described within the traditional medical model. The assumption is that they are therapeutic and the basis of evaluation is successful treatment, in this case a pregnancy or a child. Second, they fulfill a couple's desire to have a family, which is a powerful cultural value. Third, the birth technologies are a way to help individuals exercise their reproductive rights. Thus the technologies enhance freedom and enable rights to be exercised, thereby helping to fulfill two of our most significant cultural values. Fourth, physicians have typically enjoyed significant freedom of professional action. They are correctly perceived as wanting to benefit patients, and society has allowed physicians considerable latitude in decision making. Finally, the birth technologies are yet another example of the wonders and marvels of modern science and medicine. And to reject these, one would apparently also have to reject progress, our most highly valued product.

Thus it should come as no surprise that few people have

stepped back and conducted a technological assessment. In typical American fashion, we have allowed the technology to develop in advance of any examination or evaluation of it or its potential implications. Our cultural bias for freedom and individual rights took precedence over the protection of individuals and society. It is no wonder that little, if any, attention was paid to the instruction's critique of technology and the technological imperative. Our culture is so captivated by technology and its real or imagined benefits that we are frequently blind and deaf to critiques of it, even though such critiques may be appropriate and/or necessary.

Particular attention should be paid to the instruction's insistence that research and its applications are not morally neutral and that

> one cannot derive criteria for guidance from mere technical efficiency, from research's possible usefulness to some at the expense of others, or, worse still, from prevailing ideologies.[69]

This warning is especially critical not only because of the rapidity with which new developments are made but also because of the immediacy of their application. Given high media attention to technical developments, the desire to secure a profit from one's investment, and consumer interest, an almost superhuman effort is required to ensure appropriate evaluation of the technology and its applications. This difficulty does not, however, remove the moral obligation to ensure the safety and efficacy of the technology.

Such statements are not to be interpreted as anti-technology or the product of an anti-scientific attitude. The instruction, for example, recognizes that both basic and applied research are a ". . . significant expression of this dominion of man over creation."[70] They are valuable and can promote the full flowering of humanity when directed to the benefit of all and when placed at the service of humanity. Science and technology, however, ". . . cannot of themselves show the meaning of existence and human progress."[71]

This word of caution is functionally absent from all the other documents reviewed. Appropriate words about risks and benefits will be found and suitable cautionary statements are made, and the need for research is duly noted. Most of these cautionary remarks, however, are directed to the individual utilizing the technology. The documents do not suggest, for example, how to analyze or evaluate long-term social effects. Thus, while the other documents duly sound the ritual words of caution, there are no serious provisions for a continuous analysis of the birth technologies, much less any means of curbing them in the event that problems are discovered. It is interesting to note that even the almost insurmountable problems raised by the Whitehead–Stern surrogacy case have failed to dampen people's enthusiasm for this solution to childlessness. Surely the instruction is correct when it quotes *Gaudium et Spes:*

> Our era needs such wisdom more than bygone ages if the discoveries made by man are to be further humanized. For the future of the world stands in peril unless wiser people are forthcoming.[72]

Specific Problems

Because the technologies are relatively recent, a number of problems have not yet been resolved, although their existence surfaced almost as soon as the technologies were applied.

The first of these is the issue of to whom the technologies are available. The critical subissues here are cost and class. The procedure is expensive, costs will remain high, and many attempts are needed to obtain a pregnancy and live birth. Even though some insurance plans are now covering IVF, a certain level of disposable income in necessary to access the clinics, especially the more successful ones.

The media or professional journals have yet to report on the birth of the first black, Hispanic, or other minority IVF baby in the United States. No members of minority groups appear to have contracted surrogates to bear children for them—nor have they been solicited as surrogate mothers. These groups may be utilizing these technologies, but there is no mention of this in the popular or professional literature.

As of now, the birth technologies are available primarily on a fee-for-service basis. Until that is resolved, there may be an inherent class and financial bias in defining the consumers of these technologies.

Second, the majority of clinics appear to provide the technologies to heterosexual married couples. There appear to be a sizeable number of gays and lesbians who would like to be parents and for whom these technologies would solve the problem of heterosexual reproduction. The general discussion of homosexuality and lesbianism is already a complex and difficult social issue. Making these technologies available to this group would significantly complicate this discussion. Yet if reproduction or access to it is based on the right of privacy and unless society wishes to devise and implement criteria for parenthood, the exclusion of gays and lesbians from clinics may be inappropriate, if not impossible.[73]

Similar issues are raised when single heterosexuals wish to have a child by one of these technologies. The cultural norm has been a two-parent family, though the exceptionally high divorce rate has challenged that standard. Nevertheless, the single-parent family is perceived as an exception to the cultural mores. What happens when individuals wish to make this an option, if not the norm?

Third, the issue of whether or not these technologies should be covered by insurance needs to be resolved. If, for example, the birth technologies are essentially considered as a medical treatment for infertility, then there may be no good reason why they should not be treated like any other medical treatment. But if they are seen as optional or voluntary, then the insurance question becomes a little more difficult. Some companies are covering some costs of some procedures, but not all are and certainly not all employers are making such provisions.

Attempts to resolve this question raise, of course, other serious questions: the allocation of resources, is infertility a disease, is there a right to have a child, what is society's responsibility in this, should all subscribers to an insurance plan bear the cost of reimbursement for the birth technologies? Such questions will continue to plague this discussion, but they need to be answered.

CONCLUSION

This review of various sets of guidelines on artificial reproduction shows both a diversity of value perspectives and a wide range of resolutions of the many dilemmas associated with these technologies. Other issues also lurk in the background waiting to be addressed.

A major difficulty is that the various guidelines represent a patchwork approach to the problems raised by the birth technologies. Partly this is true because there simply is no one accepted moral perspective available as the basis for an analysis of the technologies. Also determining the appropriate spokespersons to address the issues is somewhat difficult. Assumedly the group must be interdisciplinary, but what is its authority and whence is it derived? Then too if the guidelines come from a profession, their authority is limited to that profession; but such guidelines may also be biased by the interests of that profession. Finally, we need to come to terms with the fact that what the majority wants or sees as good or desirable may in fact be problematic or socially disruptive in the long run. Thus the question of appropriate legislation may conflict with people's deepest desires.

Taken as a whole, the various sets of guidelines indicate the need for some type of overview and monitoring of the various reproductive technologies. While one set may be too liberal for some and another set too conservative for others, together the various guidelines acknowledge the profound impact the birth technologies are having on individuals and the communities in which they live and acknowledge the value of a structured and restrained approach to these interventions into one of the most profound of human experiences.

5.

The Instruction as Roman Catholic Moral Teaching

The Vatican instruction on technologies to enhance the human capacity for reproduction presents a further opportunity to consider some of the assets and liabilities of the Catholic tradition of sexual ethics that was outlined in chapter 2. Chief among the issues posed by the document are: the intricacy of the method of Catholic moral theology, especially if understood as a "natural-law" method; the difficulty or at least complexity of moving from general principles to persuasively presented specific conclusions in the area of sexuality and parenthood; and the relation of Catholic teaching to social consensus and to the formation of public policy, especially in the American cultural context.

FOUNDATIONS OF THE ARGUMENT

Virtually all Christian moral teaching, including Catholic teaching, will make some reference to *scripture,* to the theological *tradition* that mediates and interprets the insights of scripture, to *philosophical* (not specifically religious) understandings of the meaning of human being and action, and to descriptive or *empirical* information about actual human experiences, communities, or activities. Christian perspectives on the moral life vary precisely in relation to the degree of emphasis or priority they give to each of these resources. It is scarcely possible to consider one in isolation from the others or to eliminate one entirely from consideration. Even if it may be claimed that "scripture alone" provides the norm of the Christian life, or that "human nature" or "Church teaching" is a sufficient basis of moral values, the other sources will converge as a sort of lens through which the evidence of the chosen source is read. But what gives a moral perspective its distinctive flavor is the fundamental importance given a particular source or sources, explicitly or implicitly.

The instruction, consistently with Catholic moral tradition, bases its key principles and arguments on a notion of human nature (especially sexual nature) expressed in the modern, personalist language of "special nature of the human person," "dignity of the human person," "sacredness of human life," "inalienable rights" and "integral good" of the human person.[1] The crucial question thus becomes how to fill out and give substance to terms such as "dignity," "rights," and "good." The cultural experiences and presuppositions, religious commitments, and scientific information available to the interpreter must and should influence the concrete meanings given to general ideals. Particularly in the realm of specific sexual and procreative acts, the foundation in "natural law" cannot remain at the level of abstract principle. It must be determined which among specific procreative options are morally acceptable in practice and in relation to the concrete circumstances that make some options possible but not others.

A basic message of the Vatican document is that moral norms cannot be derived from existential realities alone. The instruction does consider empirical information about available techniques and about the suffering of infertile couples. These realities must be evaluated in the light of values that transcend particular problems and their possible solutions. "No biologist or doctor can reasonably claim, by virtue of his scientific competence, to be able to decide on people's origin and destiny." As we have seen, the guiding values are to be the reasonable, shared ones of sex, love, procreation, and individual dignity.

These values are supported by, and often expressed in terms of, biblical and religious language such as "creature of God," "image" of God, "design and will of God," and the call to a "beatific communion" with God. But faith is not said to *add* moral obligations for Christians that ought not also be self-evident to other right-thinking people. However—and this is a crucial step in the document's method—basic human values are translated from the level of general exhortation to that of specific application by means of the guidance of previous teachings of the Catholic Church. "The Church's Magisterium . . . intends to put forward, by virtue of its evangelical mission and apostolic duty, the moral teaching corresponding to the dignity of the person and to his or her integral vocation."

As an "instruction," the document has a delimited place within the hierarchy of teaching statements of the Church. It is not "infallible" or absolutely irrevocable, but exerts a claim of serious and obedient attention on the part of Catholics especially. An overview of the various genres of Catholic teaching documents, published by the Canon Law Society of America, defines an "instruction" as "a very common form of prouncement by the Roman Curia," one which is "a doctrinal explanation, or a set of rules, directive norms, recommendations and admonitions." Instructions do not "have the force of universal laws and definitions," but are issued in order "to interpret law that is clear, not dubious." A different form of statement, the "declaration," has as its purpose "a reply to a contested point of law." In the case either of an instruction or a declaration, "their application certainly allows for more leeway than in the case of a decree."[2] Yet for this very reason, they pose difficulties of interpretation. Especially in the case of an instruction the assumption is that the relevant basic law is not disputed. Here, this basic law might be stated either in terms of the essential relation of sex, love, and parenthood or, more narrowly, as the unity of sex, love, and procreation in "each and every act." In either case, this law is simply to be applied to the case of reproductive technologies. Nothing new is added to the basic principle. If it is the narrower version of the law that is thought to be clear and uncontested, however, difficulties arise, not only because there may be doubt about whether certain techniques (e.g., GIFT, LTOT) really interfere unjustifiably with the unity of the act, but also because, in fact, the narrower statement of the law presupposed by the instruction is controverted widely.

The central teaching of the document involves the value of human life from conception and the intrinsic purposes of marriage. This value and these purposes are assumed to be grounded in natural law but are clarified in religious terms. "God alone is the Lord of life from its beginning until its end: no one can, in any circumstance, claim for himself the right to destroy directly an innocent human being." And also, "Human procreation requires on the part of the spouses responsible collaboration with the fruitful love of God; the gift of human life must be actualized in marriage through the specific and exclusive acts of husband and wife, in accordance with the laws inscribed in their persons and in their union." No variation from previous teachings is to be introduced. This returns us to a central problematic of the "natural-law" method as employed within a Christian theological tradition of ethics: What defines an authoritative "natural-law" teaching, if not self-evidently reasonable argumentation about the relatively clear application of shared values? For whom is an argument persuasive if it is proposed by an ecclesiastical or religious body, and premised on that body's authority, but not so clearly on values and specific applications acknowledged as legitimate beyond the religious community?

One asset of the natural-law method when used to address social questions such as government, economic justice, and just war, is that it enables Catholics to enter into discussion with other persons and groups in even a religiously pluralistic society. The presupposition of natural-law ethics is that there are shared values and thus moral commitments that transcend religious differences. This approach to moral questions, including those that affect society as a whole, allows Catholics to influence the resolution of questions of urgent common concern. We shall return to this question of the public function of the natural-law teaching as articulated by the Catholic magisterium after having examined more closely the steps in the presentation of the teaching itself.

TECHNOLOGICAL INTERVENTION IN REPRODUCTION

Moral Theology Background

If *Humanae Vitae* is taken as a definitive recent precedent for the Catholic understanding of sexual morality, then the groundwork laid involves the interrelation of three inseparable values: sex, love, and conception. In the past, it was the sexual act that was taken as a sort of "given" in the moral analysis. The question to be posed was, Under what circumstances may sexual acts be performed? The answer of Paul VI's encyclical is that sexual acts may be performed within a loving marital commitment, and in a manner that does not preclude, by artificial means, conception as an outcome. In other words, neither love nor conception may be deliberately separated from the triad if sexual intercourse is to be morally legitimate.

Reproductive technologies represent a new problem for moral analysis in that they can separate sex not only from love, but also from procreation, since they enable conception to occur without a sexual act. The framework for deriving the answer to the moral problem remains constant in the instruction, as in previous documents: sexual intercourse must remain part of the triad if procreation, even loving procreation by spouses, is to be morally acceptable. Visible in this case, as in that of artificial contraception, is the premise that these three goods or values must be present not only within the totality of a relationship but within "each and every act." Just as it is not sufficient that a married couple act procreatively within the totality of their sexual life, while preventing conception on some occasions; so it is not sufficient that a married couple express their love sexually on many occasions, but achieve the procreative outcome of their love by a medical means that circumvents sexual union.

Furthermore, neither in the case of contraception nor in that of technologically assisted reproduction do circumstantial barriers to the ideal justify a compromise in individual cases. While "responsible parenthood" may be the goal in view, even this end does not justify a means (contraception) that has been defined as morally objectionable in itself. While the birth and nurturing of a child may be an estimable and praiseworthy end, it may not be realized by means which are, in the repeated phrase of the instruction, "morally illicit." These limits exemplify a fundamental principle in moral thinking, both philosophical and religious: even a good end does not justify an evil means.

The use of this principle in this way in these two cases rests at the tip of a very large iceberg in recent Catholic moral thought. That iceberg is an ongoing, and often inflamed and complicated, discussion of moral norms, especially norms prohibiting specific kinds of actions absolutely, that is, no matter what the circumstances.[3] This discussion gained its real momentum from the birth-control debate of the late 1960's.[4] Questions about whether the distinction between artificial means and natural "rhythm" is really all that morally important, and about whether procreation has to be tied to each act rather than to the sexual relationship, really were precipitated by the perception—based on what some couples took to be their experience—that sometimes circumstances do change the moral quality of decisions and actions. To take an extreme illustration, using contraception to avoid a life-threatening pregnancy is morally different from using it to avoid the consequences of adultery. Thus the question was posed, Is it possible to define the moral quality of actions "in the abstract," that is, apart from circumstances and no matter what circumstances might arise? Even if it is obviously *in general better* to engage in sexual intercourse and procreation "naturally," is it sometimes permissible, or even *in the concrete circumstances better,* to interfere in what nature brings about (pregnancy in the one case and infertility in the other)? At stake here is the claim, dear to the current magisterium, that it is in fact possible to formulate absolute moral norms about specific physical actions, so that these can be decided in advance to be morally excluded, no matter what unforeseeable circumstances may come about.

A contrasting viewpoint, argued by many theologians working within the broadly Catholic tradition but called "dissenters" by the official teachers, is that acts, especially sexual acts, have to be evaluated in light of human relationships and the circumstances within which those relationships take their actual texture. This contrasting approach does not represent a cohesive "school of thought," but is rather represented by many thinkers who raise questions about the best contemporary interpretation of the Catholic natural-law tradition of moral theology.

Many questions focus on the origin and function of moral norms and on the so-called "principle of double effect." This principle is a standard means, especially in recent nineteenth- and twentieth-century Catholic moral theology, for defining norms while allowing a few closely specified exceptions. The principle essentially stands for the idea that sometimes it is not possible to do good without also causing some bad effects (hence the name), and that it is sometimes permissible to do good at the expense of evil, but not always. The principle is a tool with which to make rational distinctions among cases involving actions with "double effect." It has four conditions that set limits on the permissibility of causing evil along with good. When the conditions are met the evil caused is not moral evil, because it is not intended for its own sake and it is not out of proportion to the good accomplished. The conditions are that the act be neutral or good in itself, that is, not "intrinsically evil"; that the evil effect be tolerated only, not deliberately intended; that the evil effect not be the means to the good effect; and that the good be equal to or outweigh the evil.

The "revisionist" thinkers dispute whether the first and fundamental condition makes sense, since it may not be possible to define the evilness or goodness of actions unless circumstances are considered as well. Instead they focus on the last condition as most important, and inquire whether this is not really the gist of the principle. If so, then perhaps the first three conditions become superfluous or at least difficult to explain coherently. This explorative question-asking is not without its own practical and logical problems, and it does not amount to a "theory" as such, particularly since the questioners are not all asking or arguing the same thing. Nonetheless, the revisionists are often put into one category by virtue of the fact that they disagree with current Church teaching on one or more specific moral conclusions. They are called—usually by detractors—"proportionalists."[5] This term derives from the focus on the last condition of double effect, "proportionate reason," and is used to imply that the dissenters from the traditional interpretation are really utilitarians at heart, willing to justify any moral evil in order bring about a greater number of good consequences.

But the real issue is exactly what constitutes a "moral" evil. Perhaps some of the acts traditionally called "intrinsic evils" are evil only in a limited sense, in the sense of being compromises with imperfect or tragic circumstances. Sometimes "moral evil" or "sin" is distinguished from "nonmoral evil" or "disvalue." The latter terms refer to some unfortunate effect of an act good on the whole, an effect which is not sinful because justifiable within a whole complex of circumstances out of which the action is chosen. To return to the discussion of procreation, the instruction can be understood at one level as a reply to this intramural debate over whether artificial prevention or causation of conception is simply sinful by definition, or whether it is an unfortunate but not sinful necessity, given the limitations of situations in which some married couples may find themselves. The instruction decisively affirms the former position.

Reflected in the instruction are several of the continuing issues in understanding natural-law thinking within Catholicism. There is more at work in the derivation of conclusions than simple rational analysis or logical progression from first principles to their practical requirements. As John T. Noonan has shown,[6] historical contextualization is at least as important as reason, and certainly scripture, in determining the values and applications that will be stressed in relation to Catholic sexual morality. The document on procreation is responding to cultural trends regarding sex and parenthood, trends perceived as dangerous to the family and the unborn; to rapid developments in medical technology that may be equally dangerous; and also to debates within Catholicism over positions that are perceived by some as markers of loyalty or disloyalty to the Church. The emphasis on the importance of adherence to traditional values and teachings, and on the responsibilities of the Church to teach and clarify the natural law, are a means to foreclose debate over controverted moral positions, and to disallow the possibility that logically flawed or experientially unverified arguments on behalf of some teachings are adequate cause for doubting their authority.

Artificial Fertilization

The emphasis in this discussion is on the place of procreation within marriage. The first topic to be addressed is heterologous artificial fertilization, which is rejected because "The fidelity of the spouses in the unity of marriage involves reciprocal respect of their right to become a father and a mother only through each other." There is also appeal to a "right" of the child to be conceived, born, and brought up within marriage. The place of all "truly responsible procreation" in marriage is confirmed both by the "tradition of the Church" and by "anthropological reflection."[7] Put negatively, recourse to a third person "constitutes a violation of the reciprocal commitment of the spouses," of the "unity" of the marriage, and of the "rights of the child."[8]

Although artificial insemination and *in vitro* fertilization within the marriage bond do not interrupt the unity of the marriage bond itself, or the unity of marital and parental love, they are rejected on the basis of the arguments put forward in *Humanae Vitae* and by John Paul II in his reaffirmations of it. "Such fertilization is neither in fact achieved nor positively willed as the expression and fruit of a specific act of the conjugal union."[9] Moreover, a child "is not an object to which one has a right," rather "a child is a gift." Despite the significant and tragic suffering of infertile couples, whose desire for a child is quite legitimate, the implementation of artificial means of conception violates the dignity of the child to be, as well as their commitment as spouses, and the meaning of marital sexuality.[10] It is not clarified why rejecting the idea that parenthood is a "right," and affirming the idea that children are a "gift," precludes intervention in order to bring that "gift" about. The idea that the births of children should be left entirely up to Divine Providence is negated by Paul VI's affirmation of "responsible parenthood," that is, of a proper place for human intervention in family size and the spacing of children. Certainly the Church does not reject *all* medical attempts to enhance fertility and produce pregnancy, nor, for that matter, to avoid it. So intervention as such is not the issue. The "right" versus "gift" rhetoric seems more properly to get at the problem of proper attitudes toward children and toward the parental role, rather than at choice of means to create that role. The question not completely answered is where and why the line should be drawn in distinguishing morally acceptable means of seeking a child from those which are morally objectionable.

Interestingly, the instruction's discussion of homologous fertilization contains a qualification by which it is differentiated morally from methods using donors. A method used in marriage, even though "in itself illicit," "is not marked by all that ethical negativity found in extra-conjugal procreation; the family and marriage continue to constitute the setting for the birth and upbringing of the children."[11] Against the background of traditional Catholic teaching, this constitutes a rather remarkable statement. In the first place, the tradition made no distinctions of gravity among sexual sins; all were considered "mortal." The end result was that everything from contraception and masturbation to adultery and rape were treated simply as "intrinsically evil," and any contemplation of possible exceptions to the rule was precluded.[12] Not only is a distinction made, but it is linked to the *relationships* in which the "illicit" acts are carried out or which they make possible. This represents another move away from the individual-act-centered view of sexual and procreative morality, although the specific action-guiding rule remains directed to the sexual nature and procreative openness of "each and every act."

The methodological aim of the instruction seems to be to appeal to a consensus on the meaning of marriage, sex, and parenthood, a consensus built from the experience of married persons and parents, articulated through reasonable philosophical reflection on the values concerned, and clarified by the tradition and teaching of the Catholic Church. The fundamental problem that can arise for such a method is that what it presumes to be a relative consensus on the matters it addresses may not exist. In offering its "reasonable" analysis, the document draws largely on the general Thomistic tradition, with its respect for ordered community and social interdependence; hierarchical values and authorities that delineate them; and its reliance on physical nature and basic natural relationships as the stuff out of which moral norms can be fashioned. Its arguments may be unconvincing to those who share a different worldview, one with which the document does not fully reckon and in regard to whose insights and persuasive power the document seems almost naïve. If the arguments offered do not persuade, then a consensus will not be created, unless those to whom the appeal is made accept Church authority, with or without supporting reasons.

The other worldview in competition with that of the document is one with which modern Catholic thought has made an uneasy alliance by employing the rhetoric of individual dignity, freedom, love, and rights to bolster its standard conclusions. Perhaps not seen clearly is the fact that this language can be grounded in a view of the human being and of human values that is in some ways at odds with the Catholic, Thomistic one. In Western, post-Enlightenment, democratic cultures the prime values are the freedom and equality of the individual, his or her autonomy and privacy, and the importance of free agreement or contract in creating or dissolving moral obligations. Civil society and especially government exist in order to enhance freedom as far as possible by ensuring that the freedoms of one person or group do not infringe unfairly on those of others. It is difficult to find a place in such a world for "natural" duties arising out of relationships—much less physical processes—that were not chosen or at least accepted by the individual person. Statements to the effect that the "unity" of marriage or the "dignity" of spouses and offspring precludes procreative agreements with third parties—much less control of the physical reproductive event—will fall on deaf ears.

Why should not the "dignity" of spouses simply require that both be respectful of the serious needs and choices of the other, and that no decision be taken without the fully considered and complete agreement of both? Why should not the "unity" of marriage mean that neither partner would undertake to procreate a child without the other's wholehearted consent, and that both would share equally in the loving upbringing of the child? Why does the "dignity of the procreation of the human person" preclude a surrogate-mother role for a woman who acts out of altruistic motives, who knows that the couple to raise her child want it desperately, and can reasonably be expected to be responsible and loving parents? The authors of the instruction may be inadequately attuned to the fact that their *statements* about what marriage and parenthood require do not constitute *arguments,* especially for those who do not share their basic frame of reference. This includes many Catholics who may look to the Church for guidance, but are also committed enough both to the Western norm of individual intelligence and responsibility and to the Catholic commitment to an objective and reasonable moral order, to reject magisterial conclusions devoid of arguments whose reasoning they can follow.

THE EMBRYO

On the question of protection of the embryo in relation to
IVF procedures, it may be that there is greater agreement
with the document within the American Catholic community,
but less agreement outside it. The Catholic Church's "pro-
life" witness in the midst of a basically pro-choice culture has
caused less division within the Church than the controversy
over contraception.[13] In our libertarian culture as a whole,
however, the Catholic abortion stance has been a source of
great resistance to the involvement of religious institutions
in public affairs. A key point distinguishing the abortion debate from that about most reproductive technologies is that
in the latter event, the individuals who choose to use the
technique may act immorally, but they do not necessarily
cause grave, immediate danger to others.

Obviously, this is not true in the abortion choice, if one
grants that the zygote, embryo, or fetus has any significant
status within the human community, and thus some moral
right to protection from harm. Even many who are not convinced that the human individual has *from conception* a full
"right to life" are skeptical of the right of its mother, given
legal protection by the 1973 Supreme Court abortion decision,
to choose to destroy it on behalf of any interest of her own,
up to the point of viability and perhaps further. The status
of the fetus assumed in U.S. abortion policy is not entirely
consistent with the policy recommendations on infertility
therapies that were outlined in chapter 4.[14] This fact inclines
to substantiate a potential consensus that, while the embryo
is not to be treated as the equivalent of a "baby," neither
should it be viewed and disposed of as mere "tissue." Furthermore, federal restrictions on the use of fetuses in research
tends to support the view that attitudes toward human life
even in its earliest and, to some, "prepersonal" stages have

implications for respect for human life generally, and that trivialization of the value of the first can erode social policies of protection for the second. While agreement may not be forthcoming for the position that even the fertilized egg, blastocyst, and zygote should be regarded as having the dignity of a human person, the warning of the document that "techniques of fertilization *in vitro* can open the way to other forms of biological and genetic manipulation of human embryos" does not lack persuasive power.

The physician and humanist philosopher Leon Kass cautioned, after the birth of Louise Brown, that while there is no intrinsic objection to IVF within marriage, "there will almost certainly be other uses, involving third parties . . .,"[15] To use a "surrogate womb," in another third-party relation to an infertile couple, is to treat the body "as a mere incubator, divested of its human meaning. It is also to deny the meaning of the bond among sexuality, love, and procreation."[16] Kass projects long-term laboratory growth of embryos, genetic experimentation on embryos, and the commercial banking of embryos.[17] As he points out, there are two different sorts of concerns involved in analyzing the morality of acts and practices, including procreative ones. The first and most obvious is the *intrinsic* rightness or wrongness of the case immediately at hand. The second is the likely *consequences* of performing an act or instituting a practice. While possible consequences alone do not determine intrinsic morality, they must be part of the full moral consideration of decision making. Immoral consequences can follow from a justifiable act or class of acts *either* if the original justifying reasons (a "right" to have a child) could be extended from morally permissible to other and morally objectionable acts (from homologous to heterologous means, for example); *or* if social acceptance of a certain class of acts is likely to erode the social policies that limit recourse to that class alone, and thus to prepare the way for new and less morally acceptable practices (from IVF to experimentation on the embryo and fetus).

AMERICAN RECEPTION

The Vatican's instruction on human life and procreation received an unusual amount of notice in the American press. *The New York Times* not only gave it front-page coverage and reported reactions for days following its publication, but printed the entire document.[18] The *Times* also reported international reactions, which varied in tone, but generally were not as expansive as that in the U.S.[19] Certainly the public attention concurrently given the "Baby M" surrogate mother case, then pending in New Jersey, helped make the document newsworthy in this country. Nonetheless, such attention accorded to the moral exhortations of one religious denomination remains remarkable in our pluralist and individualist society. Certainly it appears that some Americans were receptive to some reasonable and prudent analysis of the moral dilemmas posed by the galloping use of medical technologies to create children in new ways, involving innovative combinations of adults.

The *Times* presented a broad diversity of reactions to the document's conclusions. Letting the Vatican make its own case, Roberto Suro summarized its central conclusions, and quotes "chief Vatican spokesman, Joaquin Navarro-Valls," as explaining that "in this document the church was addressing a much broader audience than usual because 'it asks government leaders, be they Catholic or not, to firmly impose moral norms on certain medical and scientific activities.' "[20] Ari L. Goldman reports support for the document among American Catholic religious leaders, such as Bishop Francis J. Mugavero (Brooklyn), who welcomed the clarification offered by the statement, and promised that it would be "read and analyzed carefully for guidance within our own health-care system."[21] Yet Goldman also includes less affirmative responses from theologians whom he characterizes as "dissenting", yet "widely characterized as moderates within the spectrum of Catholic thinking in the United States." These include Richard A. McCormick, S.J., who does not find the Vatican argument "persuasive." "The document argues that a child can be born only from a sexual act. . . . The most that can be argued is that a child should be born within a marriage from a loving act. Sexual intercourse is not the only loving act."[22] Philosopher Daniel Callahan, director of the Hastings Center, pointed out the importance of "human nature" in defining Catholic moral norms. "It seems that whenever there is any deviation from natural modes of procreation . . . the Vatican has objected, arguing that any human intervention in this area is likely to be wrong and dangerous." He contrasted this approach with "extreme" views of individual freedom common in American culture, views according to which " 'human beings can do whatever they want, as long as there is no obvious palpable harm to others.' "[23] Some infertile couples, including Catholics, who did not argue overtly that any means whatsoever to a pregnancy is justifiable, still failed to find the document's interpretation of "natural" morality convincing or clarifying in terms of their own experience. Said one patient, "We're desperate. How can it be a sin if my husband's sperm is to be used to fertilize an egg from me and I give birth from my womb? I think God wants us to have children. How can that be a sin?"[24]

As Catholic theological reflection on the Vatican's position moved from the format of the daily press to that of the weekly journal these concerns were developed somewhat more systematically. Richard McCormick notes that while the contents of the instruction were hardly unexpected, neither are they a closure to the discussion, since the authors, in the conclusion, invite theologians and moralists to further consideration of the issues.[25] McCormick expresses appreciation for the attention called to "profoundly important" issues, especially "some very basic human values such as marriage, parenthood, the good of children." He notes that if all moral evaluation of reproductive technologies focuses on one objective only, "the provision of a child to a couple who cannot otherwise have one," the resulting analysis is likely to "steamroller" other key issues, such as the "runaway" and "unregulated" course of technology. Technology must be supervised, and policy that can accomplish this depends on the consensus of an informed public. But support for restraints will be forthcoming "only if the lines are drawn in the right place."

It is the drawing of specific moral lines by the instruction that is cause for most concern. When is technology dehumanizing and when is it truly at the service of the human person? How is this to be determined? The Vatican draws the line at methods that bypass natural sexual intercourse. But why should it not be drawn instead at methods that bypass the union in love and in procreation of the spouses-parents? McCormick concurs in the congregation's stipulation that " 'the procreation of a person must be the fruit of his parents' love,' " but questions the conclusion that "when a child is 'conceived as the product of an intervention of medical or biological techniques,' he cannot be 'the fruit of his parents' love.' This is a *non sequitur,* and both prospective parents and medical technologists would recognize it as such."

Two fundamental questions of ethical analysis are implied by this exchange. First, how are arguments about what "nature" requires to be validated, and how does concrete human experience fit into the process? Second, what is the moral status of actions that fall short of the ideal, that do not fulfill essential human values to the highest degree? Certainly "natural," unobstructed intercourse that is loving and procreative is a human value and good, if considered in general or in the abstract. But is it always a good in the concrete? Can circumstances affect the moral acceptability of acts of intercourse or acts of procreation that do not realize this value fully? Using a phrase the document employs to characterize the reproductive acts that it condemns, McCormick asks, "Is an act 'deprived of its proper perfection' necessarily morally wrong?" Reflecting the general discussion about "intrinsically evil" acts and norms prohibiting them, McCormick answers, "There are many actions, less than perfect, actions that contain positive disvalues that we regard as morally permissible in the circumstances."

What is permissible in certain circumstances would then depend on an attempt to balance goods at stake in the case at hand ("proportionate reason"). But the determination of the relative priority of competing human goods is something that it is difficult to do in the abstract, except for fairly noncontroversial generalizations, such as "life takes priority over property." There is a problem in the Vatican statement that reflects a problem both in the natural-law tradition and in the popular responses to the statement as reported in the press. This is the need to rely on human experience in gaining insight into the realms of value called into question in concrete moral dilemmas. It is experience that is supposedly the substratum of natural-law reflection; yet it is also experience that is the ground of challenges to the Vatican's insistence that sex, love, and procreation be kept together in "each and every act." On the one hand, evaluation becomes meaningless if it is cut loose from concrete experience; on the other, experience becomes directionless if it is unguided by reasonable generalizations about what would be morally praiseworthy and blameworthy in similar circumstances.

How can the problem—the role of experience in moral judgment—be resolved? In an earlier essay, McCormick offered some "unsolicited suggestions" to the authors of a Vatican document on bioethics that McCormick had learned was in the process of composition. These suggestions (now apparently unheard or unheeded) amounted to a *process* of moral consideration and clarification that might have balanced reliance on experience in the process of moral evaluation with the need to subject experience itself to some transcendent and consistent values. McCormick advised that moral discussion take place according to the traditional Catholic criterion of "reason informed by faith" (not replaced by it), and by the Vatican II criterion of human nature "integrally and adequately considered" (not limited to physical acts). Further, an open and dialogic model of composition, similar to that used by the U.S. bishops in their letter on peace and the economy, would provide a "give-and-take" between the tradition and present circumstances. This implies both that the competence of discussion-partners be taken seriously and that magisterial teaching itself be viewed as "provisional and open to revision."[26] The final product on reproductive technologies, however, seems neither to have been the result of the broad consultation it claims, nor to have proceeded from the premise that a genuinely new perspective on some of the issues might be developed through conversation with those the issues most closely involve. As *America* editorialized the document is not without reason perceived as "deductive" in its method. Before the discussion of *in vitro* fertilization for married couples is even begun, "principles" are clarified, which—it is to become clear—"ruled out beforehand the possibility of *in vitro* fertilization for married couples." Even though the document presents its arguments carefully, "there is a remarkably detached and even naïve way in which it expends its authority."[27]

The best defenders of the document—prudently and with moral legitimacy—focus not on the negative proscriptions of artificially achieved conception in marriage, but on some of the larger questions about the human meanings of sex, marriage, parenthood, technology, and the life of the species in its earliest or most vulnerable stages. Cardinal Joseph Bernardin of Chicago, in an address at the University of Chicago,[28] explained that three "principles" shape the conclusions of the instruction: the dignity of every human life; the essential relationship between human sexuality, marriage, and parenthood; and the essential relationship between "love-making and life-making" in each act of marital intercourse. Acknowledging that the third principle is the most controverted, Bernardin points out that it at least should raise the question whether the qualitative uniqueness of human intercourse calls for great caution and restraint in subjecting it to "scientific planning" and technology. Regarding the dignity of life, Bernardin acknowledges "the complexity of scientific evidence" about early development, and focuses on use of diagnostic techniques in destroying "imperfect" fetuses and on experimentation. Affirming the basic connection among sex, marriage, and parenthood, the Cardinal notes that their "essential unity" is violated by donor methods. "Although people sympathize with the desire of a couple or an individual to have a child, most are very uncomfortable with the separation of the generation of life from the stable context of married family life." Bernardin offers "love, support, and understanding" to childless couples who consider the use of scientific technology to assist conception within marriage. "And in the end, after prayerful and conscientious reflection on this teaching, they must make their own decision."

Daniel E. Pilarczyk, Archbishop of Cincinnati, repudiates pragmatic, individualist utilitarianism when he rejects the idea of a "right" to have a child, especially a right exercised through "any available means." There are some human situations, however painful, that simply must be accepted because to alter them would exact too great a moral cost. He also expresses concern about the long-range consequences of exerting unjustified control over human procreation and human life. "Even if the logical conclusions of the undertaking are not seen at the beginning, or are deliberately rejected, the logic is there, waiting for its chance to assert itself along the path on which it has been set." The Church has a responsibility to take a cautionary stand, even if unpopular.[29]

The dominant theme of James T. Burtchaell, C.S.C., is the moral necessity to limit technology in light of a modern and holistic understanding of the demands of the natural law.[30] Burtchaell astutely focuses on the point behind the concern of many that technology has about it an uncontrollability that readily escapes moral control. "The vulnerability of modern technology consists in its readiness to view tasks no more largely than the desires they are asked to satisfy." Correlatively, "the technologist is a 'can do' person whose success is usually proportionate to his or her ability to fix total attention upon a given problem, to isolate it from all extrinsic factors, and resolutely to manipulate the variables in order to produce the client's satisfaction."[31] One of the crucial insights behind the Vatican's stress on the unity of sex with both love and procreation is that sexual intercourse can be "a vital and intrinsic link" in the relation not only between spouses but between those spouses and their children. It is not only possible but "naturally necessary" for persons "to celebrate both of their most loyal commitments in sex." The unity and irrevocability of basic forms of human relationship and commitment are expressed in the act of love that also becomes an act of parenting. In such an act it is acknowledged and respected that some future choices will be foreclosed in favor of obligations already undertaken and requiring fidelity. Sexual love and procreation are not two separate objects of choice, but unified relationships whose meaning is intelligible not in isolation from one another, but only in relation to one another and to the total, faithful commitments of the persons who make them. "Technology is proposed as the instrument of human self-determination, freedom and choice, but if it is used to subvert our inherent needs and obligations, it will surely handicap and even destroy us."[32]

Burtchaell, however, does not shy away from the hard question of line-drawing, or resort to rhetoric about abuses of technology rather than argument about its proper place.

This in fact is "the gaping question Rome has not yet resolved: How *do* we discern where technology is enhancing nature? How do we discriminate between what is appropriately and inappropriately artificial?"[33] The language of "dignity of the person" calls out for substance. Burtchaell perceives one of the key principles of the document to be that "Conception may be assisted but never dominated by technical assistance." It is precisely this that would constitute a violation of human sex and conception precisely as *human* events. Yet this valid principle is not applied by the document as carefully as could be desired. In fact, the document almost seems to fall into the trap of technological thinking when it isolates the sex act from the spousal-parental relationship, and thereby encourages a "casuistry" of manipulation whereby various techniques (e.g., the perforated condom) are invented in order to preserve the integrity of the act while still achieving the desired end of alleviating infertility. Burtchaell, on the other hand, believes there may be

> good reason to consider contraception, IVF and AIH as capable of enhancing the natural course of a marital life in the same way that a Caesarean section and bottle-feeding with special supplements do. There can be artifice and technology that enhance nature. But that needs to be evaluated within the full continuity and integrity of a couple's sexual life. The moral worth of technical intervention would derive from whether the union itself was generous between the spouses and toward offspring.[34]

These are not specifically religious arguments. Burtchaell portrays the Vatican doctrine as a religiously motivated witness to what are, after all, common appreciations of the significance of sexuality within marriage and as conducive toward parenthood. It is not Catholics only who should perceive danger in a technology that neglects a vision of the whole. But, as several commentators have indicated, it is the general contours of the instruction that are convincing as cultural critique. There is more consensus behind its fundamental insights into the unity of the sex-love-procreation triad, and the necessity that a broader striving toward global values limit the problem-solution technological mentality, than there is behind its derivative moral norms.

Taking a thoughtful humanistic rather than a specifically religious stance, Charles Krauthammer demonstrates the potential of the document for credibility beyond a narrowly Catholic audience. Contrasting the Vatican declaration favorably with the British, Australian, and American Fertility Society recommendations, Krauthammer commends it as "a radical act of resistance to the technological hubris of modern reproductive medicine. . . ."[35] Three new scientific capabilities present corresponding dangers: fetal manipulation and experimentation is a threat to human dignity; third-party donation of gametes is a threat to the family; conception without sexual intercourse is a threat to sexuality. And yet, objects Krauthammer, the document forfeits effectiveness because it "opposes everything"—not content with sand-bagging the slippery slope, the Church "declares the entire mountain off-limits."[36] The result is practical vacuousness: "Too many fences make for none."[37] If civil society is to be convinced in favor of social policies that discourage third-party involvements such as the use of surrogate mothers, then a more serious "moral calculus" is needed, one that can weigh the evil of infertility both against immediate abuses of the new technologies and against the risk of future increased abuse (qualitative or quantitative). "To avoid the horrors of the new reproductive science, our most important weapon may be nuance."[38] Krauthammer suggests that better places to draw lines marking off illegitimate means of remedying infertility would be at the boundary of the marriage commitment, and at the fourteen-day stage for the conceptus (roughly the time of implantation).

PARALLEL CASES

It is important to note that the instruction on reproductive technologies moves decisively to introduce into the public-policy arena its recommendations regarding matters to which, in traditional terms, reference might have been made as "personal ethics." The recent pastoral letters of the American bishops on issues of social concern have made it increasingly clear that the Catholic Church and its moral-theological tradition have had a tendency to divide the moral life into two compartments, and to adopt different and not entirely compatible models for analysis in each.

On questions of social, political, and economic organization the modern papal social encyclicals—from *Rerum Novarum* (Leo XIII, 1981) through *Pacem in Terris* (John XXIII, 1963) to *Laborem Exercens* (John Paul II, 1981)—have provided productive examples of witness to natural-law values, backed up by religious imagery, but articulated primarily in terms of "common good," "justice," "duties," "rights," and so on. A strength of these encyclicals has been that they employ one basic framework, that of the sociality of persons, each with personal dignity but intrinsically dependent on and contributing to the social fabric, which can be used flexibly to address different historical circumstances, their particular opportunities, challenges, and dangers. The Catholic witness itself has been shaped differently, depending on the perceived needs of the day, so that, e.g., socialism may be repudiated in favor of private property at one time, and at another capitalism may be criticized in favor of more equitable distribution of world resources.[39] Specific conclusions, in the sense of morally mandatory political strategies or legal enactments, are rarely put forward, and never with the force of indisputable authority. Thus the task of implementation of the ideal in particular social contexts or in view of various circumstances is left to the governments and citizens to which the appeal is addressed.

The American episcopal pastorals follow in this tradition, although with a longer and more explicitly dialogical process of drafting and critique preceding the publication of each letter. Each moves as far as possible toward policy recommendations, since the bishops perceive it as their duty as religious and moral leaders not to leave their message at the level of vague idealism. The "peace pastoral" states that the use of nuclear weapons to kill noncombatants would be immoral, suggests that nuclear deterrence is at the least morally "paradoxical" because it buys peace at the expense of threatening and even intending to do what it would be immoral to carry out, and offers criteria for evaluating the development of weapons systems within what should be a long-term project of mutual arms reduction. The economics pastoral recommends drastic revisions in the American capitalist system, so that a much lower unemployment rate would be the maximum acceptable; so that government-funded benefits for those in poverty be increased, especially benefits for female heads-of-household and their families; and so that the United States would take a more active role in alleviating such international economic crises as the Third World debt. These pastorals were envisioned by their authors as contributions to an ongoing discussion, and they invited debate. Although, in contrast to the papal encyclicals, these were contributions of the local hierarchy, they followed in the social-encyclical tradition of exhortation and admonishment, not the proscription in absolute terms of closely defined activities. They were quite successful, as were the social encyclicals, in stimulating public debate and in bringing to public attention previously submerged moral concerns regarding morally dubious social trends.

Church teaching on matters of sexual morality, and in many areas of medical morality related to sexuality, has been shaped on a different model. As we have seen, not only has the Church developed quite specific moral norms, but it has also exerted on their behalf a considerable degree of authority (e.g., calling all contrary acts "morally illicit"), and it has not invited broad consultation with an eye to revision of its proposals if need be. As unfortunately we have also seen, this approach tends to induce a response that focuses on the negative prohibitions just as quickly as did the initial statement. Finding these logically unconvincing and unconfirmed by experience, much of the audience becomes quickly disaffected, and credibility for the Church's standpoint in general is diminished seriously. It is not to be expected that a pronouncement of the magisterium would explicitly retract a statement (such as the "each and every act" analysis of *Humanae Vitae*) still quite clearly in the memory of both Catholic and non-Catholic audiences. Yet it does not seem unrealistic to expect the Church to gauge the social temperature well enough to estimate more accurately just where, when, and in what terms a socially productive moral witness can be uttered. A more effective statement might have spent its energy on the valid and important points so appreciated by McCormick, Burtchaell, and Krauthammer, and left in the background the precise implications of the analysis of *Humanae Vitae* for these new questions.

Given the statement in the form it actually did assume, a great deal of its future effectiveness will depend on its implementation. It remains possible for the interpreter to continue to stress the strong points of the document, transcending the narrower, more condemnatory language with greater success than the document itself exhibits. The local bishop, in the U.S. or elsewhere, will also have a significant role to play in educating Catholics in his diocese about the contents and significance of the document; in deciding in what style to supervise infertility programs in Catholic hospitals in his diocese; and in deciding the tone and content of presentations of Catholic teaching that are made by representatives of the diocese to non-Catholic groups and to legislators and to policy-makers. Despite the initial flurry of intense attention, local implementation will play a determining role in the long-range effect the Vatican instruction is to have. In this way, the potential for effectiveness or destructiveness of the document is similar to that of the birth-control encyclical. While that encyclical became an occasion for, and continues to be a symbol of, divisiveness within the American Church, the same need not be true of the document on reproduction. After *Humanae Vitae,* many episcopal conferences internationally moved to offer interpretive statements with the aim of enhancing its positive and decreasing its negative impact, for instance by expressing the pastoral concern of the Church or by allowing some independence for the individual conscience in the appropriation of the encyclical's mandates. Unfortunately, in the United States, the struggle between doctrinal, ecclesiastical, and liturgical conservatives and liberals found in the encyclical a perfect battleground for the differences generated or at least polarized by the rapid changes following the Council. We have in the 1980's a different ecclesial setting, in which the bishops have already led the U.S. Church in civil discussion on controversial issues and in which, at least on some issues (such as "abortion on demand"), relatively liberal and relatively conservative Catholics have already managed to forge alliances against dominant cultural mores. There can still exist hope that this Vatican instruction will provoke and not preclude thoughtful self-criticism within modern Western and Catholic culture.

A final but important factor in the North American cultural context is the gaining influence of Christian feminism and the rapidly changing social roles of women generally. Feminism, Catholic-identified or not, is not a movement that the Church particularly has encouraged. Nonetheless, John Paul II is at least moderately sympathetic to women's social participation and enhanced equality within the family. An opportunity for moral witness in the area of reproductive techniques arises out of the tendency of some of these either to define women's role in terms of childbearing, or to take advantage of poor women, or both. Many commentators on the "Baby M" surrogate-mother case took note of the fact that surrogates are likely to be economically and socially disadvantaged compared to their male "clients." One might also question the social and moral implications of a man's overriding need to continue his genetic line, rather than joining with his infertile partner in adopting a child related in the same way to both of them. Equality of man and woman in the spousal relationship seems fittingly represented by their mutual love for a child whom they choose to bring into their family through a relationship of parenthood that is biologically equal for both of them. Adoption of a child is not morally the same either for the yielding or receiving parents as the creation of a child through ovum, sperm, or embryo donation or surrogacy. In the typical adoption case, the genetic mother or parents do not conceive a child with the explicit intention of severing all ties of the parental relationship to that child. The adoption is the result of some set of circumstances that were unforeseen, and which the parties to the adoption would agree were originally unfortunate. Adoption is a responsible intervention into those unplanned circumstances, bringing out of it a new set of relationships that will best serve the dignity and welfare of birth parents, adoptive parents, and child. The same holds in the case of a spouse who adopts the already existing children of his or her marriage partner.

The negative moral implications of asserting an overriding need for or right to a genetic bond with one's "own" child is not a feminist issue alone, of course, since much the same as above could be suggested of a woman who uses a sperm donor if her husband is infertile. In the latter case, however, the need expressed is usually not so clearly for continuation of the blood line, but the woman's strong desire to be pregnant and "carry her own child." Does this imply that a woman's truest fulfillment is in childbearing, or that her status and value in life is determined by her ability to do this? This was the mindset with which Sarah resorted to encouraging a "surrogate" pregnancy begun by her husband Abraham with her maid Hagar (Gen. 16). Not only did this have divisive and tragic circumstances for all concerned (Gen. 21), but it represents an attitude toward the all-importance of genetic kinship that is decisively set aside in the ministry of Jesus and his first followers.

The procreative relationship of parent to child is undeniably a great and precious good. But it is not an absolute value, one which should be sought at any cost and through any means. The love commitment of spouses sets reasonable, humane, and Christian parameters in which to undertake parenthood. Even within marriage, the use of technology should be judged in relation to the love and commitment of spouses, and by its effects on their relationship. It seems reasonable to ask whether the stress and frustration associated with use of reproductive therapies may sometimes be disproportionate, given their low success rate. As Burtchaell indicates, the pitfall of technology is precisely a narrowing of focus to a problem and its possible solution, so that a proper view of the whole within which the solution makes sense is lost. This is not to preclude in advance all use of reproductive technologies, especially as their success rate is improved. A basic point of the Vatican document, however, is well-taken; procreation should not be considered as an independent objective, detached from its integral and human relation to the totality of a marital love relation.

6.

Conclusions

Through our review and analysis of reproduction therapies, we have attempted to demonstrate that moral assessment of new technical and social developments does not present an insuperable challenge to Catholic tradition, when that tradition draws on the best of its resources and addresses the present cultural situation in a sensitive manner. In the words of Cardinal Joseph Bernardin, the "natural-law" tradition represents the conviction that human experience is ordered by values and meaning that are "accessible to all people of good will who reflect with care and wisdom on the experience of life."[1] At the same time, as Bernardin also takes note, "Contemporary philosophical and sociological developments have made us more aware of the contextual nature of all knowledge. That is why it is possible that what appears to be a proper understanding or application of an ethical principle in one age may be found wanting or even incorrect in another."

In a sense, the present study is an attempt to "recontextualize" the Catholic Christian understandings of the spheres of sexual activity, parenthood, and married love. The purpose of the process has been to retrieve and renew basic human and Christian insights into these realities, and so to arrive at an improved grasp of their moral meanings, and of the possibilities and limits of morally responsible action within them. In addition to basic empirical information, Catholic ethics includes among its sources biblical understandings of women, parenthood, and marriage; philosophical ("natural-law") interpretations of normative values and principles to guide action; and past uses by key theologians and Church statements of biblical, philosophical, and empirical sources ("tradition"). Within these resources are visible both lines of continuity and of change in Catholic views of sexuality, procreation, and marriage.

Descriptive or Empirical Accounts

Our examination began with empirical information about the available techniques, their frequency of use, and their success rates. Artificial insemination with semen either from a donor or from the husband of the recipient woman is technically and socially well established, and offers a high rate of success. This is the technique by which "surrogate mothers" are enabled to bear children for the men with whom they contract. *In vitro* fertilization and embryo transfer, on the other hand, continue to be improved scientifically but offer at present a disappointingly low chance of success for most of the couples (customarily married) to whom the process is available. Although there appears to be no significant risk to children who are born as a result of the process, questions remain about the fate of other embryos created *in vitro,* both those not chosen for implantation and those chosen for cryo-preservation. There is no uniform protocol followed by IVF programs specifying what shall be done with superfluous embryos. Perhaps more importantly, there remains the possibility that embryos may be cultivated in the laboratory, beyond the implantion stage, for the purpose of genetic and fertility research.

Committees established by secular, governmental, or professional groups generally accept AIH, AID, and IVF, but limit laboratory growth of embryos to fourteen days. They do not require that all embryos be implanted. While some reservations are expressed about surrogate motherhood, owing to contractual uncertainties, lack of social acceptance, and deleterious psychological effects on the child (especially when she or he becomes the subject of a dispute), moratoria on the practice appear provisional rather than absolute. Neither the destruction of the zygote or early embryo, nor "third-party" or donor methods of procreation have as such been portrayed as objectionable on moral grounds by most policy committees, nor by many individual social commentators outside the Catholic tradition.

Included within the empirical or "factual" category is a somewhat looser description and prediction of the sociocultural effects of the relevant technologies. It seems hard to deny that, at the least, the pain of childlessness plus the availability of medical remedies and the libertarian Western ethos combine to support an atmosphere of social and legal permissiveness toward those who, in order to produce the children so strongly desired, contract with medical professionals and with fertile individuals who can provide sperm, ova, embryos, or wombs. Those arguing in favor of such contracts might well appeal to the "right to reproductive self-determination" already well supported by U.S. abortion policy, although the status of this right is still debated, and even such a right may not confer the right to have a child. While most other documents to date have welcomed reproduction technologies with few limits, the Vatican document and its supportive interpreters sound a much more cautious note.

Scripture

From the Hebrew Bible the Christian tradition receives a high respect for parenthood and for the gift of children. Would-be parents such as Abraham, Sarah, Jacob, and Rachel hardly leave the creation of the child up to the will of God, however. In offering their husbands "surrogates" for their own fertility, these women sought to verify their own womanhood and to make their contribution as wives and as mothers of sons to the continuation of the family and of the Chosen People. On the negative side must be counted the competition and strife among wives, surrogates, and their offspring; and the assumption that the role of women (and of sexual intercourse) consists above all else in childbearing. The Genesis creation accounts offer in critical counterpoint a vision of male and female united equally for parenthood and for social partnership, and of sexuality as expressing that unity in "one flesh." In the New Testament, the all-important function of family in determining religious identity is set aside, and with it the Israelite significance of sex, marriage, and parenthood. This shift is especially noteworthy in regard to the role of women. Women are included in important religious roles in Jesus's ministry and in the mission of the early Church, and these are not tied to their spousal and maternal roles. One consequence is to reduce the significance of parenthood in defining personal identity, especially that of women. The implications of this shift have yet to be fully realized in Roman Catholic sexual ethics or social thought.

Tradition

Augustine and Aquinas absorb from dualistic philosophies the perception that physical passions are morally problematic, but also appreciate the goodness of created nature, and so justify sexual actions by directing them toward procreation. Aquinas in particular expresses this standpoint in terms of basic human purposes and values, saying that it is a requirement of the natural law that each species should procreate itself. Humans, with reason and free will, should respect this natural inclination, and also the natural structure of the physical act by which procreation takes place. The procreative focus for sexuality has remained a prominent characteristic of the Christian tradition, although it has been accompanied by a latent appreciation that sex has a positive relation to the love of spouses and to their partnership across all spheres of life. Aquinas spoke of the "friendship" of spouses. At the time of the Second Vatican Council, Catholic teaching was reformulated specifically to include both love and procreation as intrinsic purposes of sexuality. The encyclical *Humane Vitae* ties these values to "each and every act" of sexual intercourse, prohibiting contraception and likewise implying the prohibition of fertilization without sexual intercourse. It is this conclusion that the recent instruction makes explicit and which serves as the basis for much discussion of Roman Catholic sexual ethics.

Current Philosophical Reflection on Experience

We affirm the basic message of the instruction, which we understand to be the fundamental unity of married love, sexual expression, and openness to children. We also recognize that this unity is one that does not come into being merely as the result of human choice, but which is rooted in the human meanings of the realities themselves. It is this recognition of a basic consistency in human moral experience—not only as free and rational but also as embodied and affective—that above all else characterizes the natural-law tradition. Sexual intercourse is a "natural" expression of the committed love of a woman and a man; generally speaking, the action has an intrinsic or "natural" potential for the birth of children who become part of the love relationship of the parents.

It is dubious, however, that the experience of married persons, parents or not, clearly warrants the assertion that the love which their sexual relationship expresses must be incompatible both with occasional artifical avoidance of conception and with the use of artificial means to bring about conception without a sexual act. It is the committed love relationship of the couple in its totality that gives the moral texture both to their sexuality and to their subsequent roles as parents. It is from the wholeness of the relationship that their specific physical acts of sex and conception take their moral purpose. For the same reason, it is most consistent with the Christian and human experience of the marital bond to protect the sexual and parental relationship of the couple within the limits of that bond. Donor methods, even when undertaken with an attitude of love toward one's spouse and one's child-to-be, allow the goal of a child genetically related to oneself to override what is properly the more fundamental commitment to sexual and procreational union with one's marriage partner, although the authors recognize that further discussion may be necessary to clarify this point.

The Vatican's call for legal prohibition of all reproduction technologies that eliminate sexual intercourse extends further than is morally necessary. From a practical standpoint, a comprehensive ban is not supported by a public consensus in the West, and would be neither feasible nor enforceable. The negative critique may, however, sound a useful warning against uncritical pursuit of that which science offers. Specifically, the critique should be articulated in the public realm in a manner focusing attention on the more morally problematic and socially objectionable practices, such as those involving parties beyond the marital union of the would-be parents. If the law should not or cannot prohibit such agreements, it may still stop short of sanctioning them by means of a legal framework that validates and protects them.

Quite obviously, these conclusions, like those of the Vatican instruction, depend on an interpretation of basic human experiences and of their moral significance. It is not possible to "prove" the validity of either set of conclusions with empirical data, philosophical argumentation, or even consistency with a religious tradition that has never before addressed precisely these questions in these circumstances; yet interaction of all these resources is vital to ongoing adequate interpretation. These areas of human moral interdependence and responsibility can be approached and understood only by contact, exchange, and argument among those who experience them and seek to understand them reasonably and in good faith. We intend our reflections to be a contribution to such exchange. We commend the method of ecumenical, interdisciplinary, and critical dialogue to all Christians who seek better to understand and persuasively to articulate the moral meaning of human procreation in the contexts of love, of love's sexual expression, and of respect for human life.

APPENDIX

Instruction on Respect for Human Life in Its Origin and on the Dignity of Procreation

FOREWORD

The Congregation for the Doctrine of the Faith has been approached by various episcopal conferences or individual bishops, by theologians, doctors and scientists, concerning biomedical techniques which make it possible to intervene in the initial phase of the life of a human being and in the very processes of procreation and their conformity with the principles of Catholic morality. The present instruction, which is the result of wide consultation and in particular of a careful evaluation of the declarations made by episcopates, does not intend to repeat all the church's teaching on the dignity of human life as it originates and on procreation, but to offer, in the light of the previous teaching of the magisterium, some specific replies to the main questions being asked in this regard.

The exposition is arranged as follows: An introduction will recall the fundamental principles of an anthropological and moral character which are necessary for a proper evaluation of the problems and for working out replies to those questions; the first part will have as its subject respect for the human being from the first moment of his or her existence; the second part will deal with the moral questions raised by tech-

140

nical interventions on human procreation; the third part will offer some orientations on the relationships between moral law and civil law in terms of the respect due to human embryos and fetuses★ and as regards the legitimacy of techniques of artificial procreation.

INTRODUCTION

1. Biomedical Research and the Teaching of the Church

The gift of life which God the Creator and Father has entrusted to man calls him to appreciate the inestimable value of what he has been given and to take responsibility for it: This fundamental principle must be placed at the center of one's reflection in order to clarify and solve the moral problems raised by artificial interventions on life as it originates and on the processes of procreation.

Thanks to the progress of the biological and medical sciences, man has at his disposal ever more effective therapeutic resources; but he can also acquire new powers, with unforeseeable consequences, over human life at its very beginning and in its first stages. Various procedures now make it possible to intervene not only in order to assist, but also to dominate the processes of procreation. These techniques can enable man to "take in hand his own destiny," but they also expose him "to the temptation to go beyond the limits of a reasonable dominion over nature."[1] They might constitute progress in the service of man, but they also involve serious risks. Many people are therefore expressing an urgent appeal that in in-

---

★The terms *zygote, pre-embryo, embryo* and *fetus* can indicate in the vocabulary of biology successive stages of the development of a human being. The present instruction makes free use of these terms, attributing to them an identical ethical relevance, in order to designate the result (whether visible or not) of human generation, from the first moment of its existence until birth. The reason for this usage is clarified by the text (cf. I, 1).

terventions on procreation the values and rights of the human person be safeguarded. Requests for clarification and guidance are coming not only from the faithful, but also from those who recognize the church as "an expert in humanity"[2] with a mission to serve the "civilization of love"[3] and of life.

The church's magisterium does not intervene on the basis of a particular competence in the area of the experimental sciences; but having taken account of the data of research and technology, it intends to put forward, by virtue of its evangelical mission and apostolic duty, the moral teaching corresponding to the dignity of the person and to his or her integral vocation. It intends to do so by expounding the criteria of moral judgment as regards the applications of scientific research and technology, especially in relation to human life and its beginnings. These criteria are the respect, defense and promotion of man, his "primary and fundamental right" to life,[4] his dignity as a person who is endowed with a spiritual soul and with moral responsibility[5] and who is called to beatific communion with God.

The church's intervention in this field is inspired also by the love which she owes to man, helping him to recognize and respect his rights and duties. This love draws from the fount of Christ's love: As she contemplates the mystery of the incarnate word, the church also comes to understand the "mystery of man";[6] by proclaiming the Gospel of salvation, she reveals to man his dignity and invites him to discover fully the truth of his own being. Thus the church once more puts forward the divine law in order to accomplish the work of truth and liberation.

For it is out of goodness—in order to indicate the path of life—that God gives human beings his commandments and the grace to observe them; and it is likewise out of goodness—in order to help them persevere along the same path—that God always offers to everyone his forgiveness. Christ has compassion on our weaknesses: He is our Creator and Redeemer. May his Spirit open men's hearts to the gift of God's peace and to an understanding of his precepts.

2. Science and Technology at the Service of the Human Person

God created man in his own image and likeness: "Male and female he created them" (Gn. 1:27), entrusting to them the task of "having dominion over the earth" (Gn. 1:28). Basic scientific research and applied research constitute a significant expression of this dominion of man over creation. Science and technology are valuable resources for man when placed at his service and when they promote his integral development for the benefit of all; but they cannot of themselves show the meaning of existence and of human progress. Being ordered to man, who initiates and develops them, they draw from the person and his moral values the indication of their purpose and the awareness of their limits.

It would on the one hand be illusory to claim that scientific research and its applications are morally neutral; on the other hand one cannot derive criteria for guidance from mere technical efficiency, from research's possible usefulness to some at the expense of others or, worse still, from prevailing ideologies. Thus science and technology require for their own intrinsic meaning an unconditional respect for the fundamental criteria of the moral law: That is to say, they must be at the service of the human person, of his inalienable rights and his true and integral good according to the design and will of God.[7]

The rapid development of technological discoveries gives greater urgency to this need to respect the criteria just mentioned: Science without conscience can only lead to man's ruin. "Our era needs such wisdom more than bygone ages if the discoveries made by man are to be further humanized. For the future of the world stands in peril unless wiser people are forthcoming."[8]

3. Anthropology and Procedures in the Biomedical Field

Which moral criteria must be applied in order to clarify the problems posed today in the field of biomedicine? The answer to this question presupposes a proper idea of the nature of the human person in his bodily dimension.

For it is only in keeping with his true nature that the human person can achieve self-realization as a "unified totality";[9] and this nature is at the same time corporal and spiritual. By virtue of its substantial union with a spiritual soul, the human body cannot be considered as a mere complex of tissues, organs and functions, nor can it be evaluated in the same way as the body of animals; rather it is a constitutive part of the person who manifests and expresses himself through it.

The natural moral law expresses and lays down the purposes, rights and duties which are based upon the bodily and spiritual nature of the human person. Therefore this law cannot be thought of as simply a set of norms on the biological level; rather it must be defined as the rational order whereby man is called by the Creator to direct and regulate his life and actions and in particular to make use of his own body.[10]

A first consequence can be deduced from these principles: An intervention on the human body affects not only the tissues, the organs and their functions, but also involves the person himself on different levels. It involves, therefore, perhaps in an implicit but nonetheless real way, a moral significance and responsibility. Pope John Paul II forcefully reaffirmed this to the World Medical Association when he said:

"Each human person, in his absolutely unique singularity, is constituted not only by his spirit, but by his body as well. Thus, in the body and through the body, one touches the person himself in his concrete reality. To respect the dignity of man consequently amounts to safeguarding this identity of the man *'corpore et anima unus,'* as the Second Vatican

Council says (*Gaudium et Spes*, 14.1). It is on the basis of this anthropological vision that one is to find the fundamental criteria for decision making in the case of procedures which are not strictly therapeutic, as, for example, those aimed at the improvement of the human biological condition."[11]

Applied biology and medicine work together for the integral good of human life when they come to the aid of a person stricken by illness and infirmity and when they respect his or her dignity as a creature of God. No biologist or doctor can reasonably claim, by virtue of his scientific competence, to be able to decide on people's origin and destiny. This norm must be applied in a particular way in the field of sexuality and procreation, in which man and woman actualize the fundamental values of love and life.

God, who is love and life, has inscribed in man and woman the vocation to share in a special way in his mystery of personal communion and in his work as Creator and Father.[12] For this reason marriage possesses specific goods and values in its union and in procreation which cannot be likened to those existing in lower forms of life. Such values and meanings are of the personal order and determine from the moral point of view the meaning and limits of artificial interventions on procreation and on the origin of human life. These interventions are not to be rejected on the grounds that they are artificial. As such, they bear witness to the possibilities of the art of medicine. But they must be given a moral evaluation in reference to the dignity of the human person, who is called to realize his vocation from God to the gift of love and the gift of life.

4. Fundamental Criteria for a Moral Judgment

The fundamental values connected with the techniques of artificial human procreation are two: the life of the human being called into existence and the special nature of the transmission of human life in marriage. The moral judgment on such methods of artificial procreation must therefore be formulated in reference to these values.

Physical life, with which the course of human life in the world begins, certainly does not itself contain the whole of a person's value nor does it represent the supreme good of man, who is called to eternal life. However it does constitute in a certain way the "fundamental" value of life precisely because upon this physical life all the other values of the person are based and developed.[13] The inviolability of the innocent human being's right to life "from the moment of conception until death"[14] is a sign and requirement of the very inviolability of the person to whom the Creator has given the gift of life.

By comparison with the transmission of other forms of life in the universe, the transmission of human life has a special character of its own, which derives from the special nature of the human person. "The transmission of human life is entrusted by nature to a personal and conscious act and as such is subject to the all-holy laws of God: immutable and inviolable laws which must be recognized and observed. For this reason one cannot use means and follow methods which could be licit in the transmission of the life of plants and animals."[15]

Advances in technology have now made it possible to procreate apart from sexual relations through the meeting *in vitro* of the germ cells previously taken from the man and the woman. But what is technically possible is not for that very reason morally admissible. Rational reflection on the fundamental values of life and of human procreation is therefore indispensable for formulating a moral evaluation of such technological interventions on a human being from the first stages of his development.

5. Teachings of the Magisterium
On its part, the magisterium of the church offers to human reason in this field too the light of revelation: The doctrine

concerning man taught by the magisterium contains many elements which throw light on the problems being faced here.

From the moment of conception, the life of every human being is to be respected in an absolute way because man is the only creature on earth that God has "wished for himself"[16] and the spiritual soul of each man is "immediately created" by God;[17] his whole being bears the image of the Creator. Human life is sacred because from its beginning it involves "the creative action of God,"[18] and it remains forever in a special relationship with the Creator, who is its sole end.[19] God alone is the Lord of life from its beginning until its end: No one can in any circumstance claim for himself the right to destroy directly an innocent human being.[20]

Human procreation requires on the part of the spouses responsible collaboration with the fruitful love of God;[21] the gift of human life must be actualized in marriage through the specific and exclusive acts of husband and wife, in accordance with the laws inscribed in their persons and in their union.[22]

I
RESPECT FOR HUMAN EMBRYOS

Careful reflection on this teaching of the magisterium and on the evidence of reason, as mentioned above, enables us to respond to the numerous moral problems posed by technical interventions upon the human being in the first phases of his life and upon the processes of his conception.

1. What respect is due to the human embryo, taking into account his nature and identity?

The human being must be respected—as a person—from the very first instant of his existence.

The implementation of procedures of artificial fertilization has made possible various interventions upon embryos and human fetuses. The aims pursued are of various kinds: diagnostic and therapeutic, scientific and commercial. From all of this, serious problems arise. Can one speak of a right to experimentation upon human embryos for the purpose of scientific research? What norms or laws should be worked out with regard to this matter? The response to these problems presupposes a detailed reflection on the nature and specific identity—the word *status* is used—of the human embryo itself.

At the Second Vatican Council, the church for her part presented once again to modern man her constant and certain doctrine according to which: "Life once conceived, must be protected with the utmost care; abortion and infanticide are abominable crimes."[23] More recently, the Charter of the Rights of the Family, published by the Holy See, confirmed that "human life must be absolutely respected and protected from the moment of conception."[24]

This congregation is aware of the current debates concerning the beginning of human life, concerning the individuality of the human being and concerning the identity of the human person. The congregation recalls the teachings found in the Declaration on Procured Abortion:

"From the time that the ovum is fertilized, a new life is begun which is neither that of the father nor of the mother; it is rather the life of a new human being with his own growth. It would never be made human if it were not human already. To this perpetual evidence . . . modern genetic science brings valuable confirmation. It has demonstrated that, from the first instant, the program is fixed as to what this living being will be: a man, this individual man with his characteristic aspects already well determined. Right from fertilization is begun the adventure of a human life, and each of its great capacities requires time . . . to find its place and to be in a position to act."[25]

This teaching remains valid and is further confirmed, if confirmation were needed, by recent findings of human biological science which recognize that in the zygote (the cell produced when the nuclei of the two gametes have fused) resulting from fertilization the biological identity of a new human individual is already constituted.

Certainly no experimental datum can be in itself sufficient to bring us to the recognition of a spiritual soul; nevertheless, the conclusions of science regarding the human embryo provide a valuable indication for discerning by the use of reason a personal presence at the moment of this first appearance of a human life: How could a human individual not be a human person? The magisterium has not expressly committed itself to an affirmation of a philosophical nature, but it constantly reaffirms the moral condemnation of any kind of procured abortion. This teaching has not been changed and is unchangeable.[26]

Thus the fruit of human generation from the first moment of its existence, that is to say, from the moment the zygote has formed, demands the unconditional respect that is morally due to the human being in his bodily and spiritual totality. The human being is to be respected and treated as a person from the moment of conception and therefore from that same moment his rights as a person must be recognized, among which in the first place is the inviolable right of every innocent human being to life.

This doctrinal reminder provides the fundamental criterion for the solution of the various problems posed by the development of the biomedical sciences in this field: Since the embryo must be treated as a person, it must also be defended in its integrity, tended and cared for, to the extent possible, in the same way as any other human being as far as medical assistance is concerned.

2. Is prenatal diagnosis morally licit?

If prenatal diagnosis respects the life and integrity of the embryo and the human fetus and is directed toward its safeguarding or healing as an individual, then the answer is affirmative.

For prenatal diagnosis makes it possible to know the condition of the embryo and of the fetus when still in the mother's womb. It permits or makes it possible to anticipate earlier and more effectively, certain therapeutic, medical or surgical procedures.

Such diagnosis is permissible, with the consent of the parents after they have been adequately informed, if the methods employed safeguard the life and integrity of the embryo and the mother, without subjecting them to disproportionate risks.[27] But this diagnosis is gravely opposed to the moral law when it is done with the thought of possibly inducing an abortion depending upon the results: A diagnosis which shows the existence of a malformation or a hereditary illness must not be the equivalent of a death sentence. Thus a woman would be committing a gravely illicit act if she were to request such a diagnosis with the deliberate intention of having an abortion should the results confirm the existence of a malformation or abnormality. The spouse or relatives or anyone else would similarly be acting in a manner contrary to the moral law if they were to counsel or impose such a diagnostic procedure on the expectant mother with the same intention of possibly proceeding to an abortion. So too the specialist would be guilty of illicit collaboration if, in conducting the diagnosis and in communicating its results, he were deliberately to contribute to establishing or favoring a link between prenatal diagnosis and abortion.

In conclusion, any directive or program of the civil and health authorities or of scientific organizations which in any way were to favor a link between prenatal diagnosis and abortion, or which were to go as far as directly to induce expectant mothers to submit to prenatal diagnosis planned for the purpose of eliminating fetuses which are affected by malformations or which are carriers of hereditary illness, is to be condemned as a violation of the unborn child's right to life and as an abuse of the prior rights and duties of the spouses.

3. Are therapeutic procedures carried out on the human embryo licit?

As with all medical interventions on patients, *one must uphold as licit procedures carried out on the human embryo which respect the life and integrity of the embryo and do not involve disproportionate risks for it, but are directed toward its healing, the improvement of its condition of health or its individual survival.*

Whatever the type of medical, surgical or other therapy, the free and informed consent of the parents is required, according to the deontological rules followed in the case of children. The application of this moral principle may call for delicate and particular precautions in the case of embryonic or fetal life.

The legitimacy and criteria of such procedures have been clearly stated by Pope John Paul II: "A strictly therapeutic intervention whose explicit objective is the healing of various maladies such as those stemming from chromosomal defects will, in principle, be considered desirable, provided it is directed to the true promotion of the personal well-being of the individual without doing harm to his integrity or worsening his conditions of life. Such an intervention would indeed fall within the logic of the Christian moral tradition."[28]

4. How is one to evaluate morally research and experimentation* on human embryos and fetuses?

Medical research must refrain from operations on live embryos, unless there is a moral certainty of not causing harm to the life or

---

*Since the terms *research* and *experimentation* are often used equivalently and ambiguously, it is deemed necessary to specify the exact meaning given them in this *integrity of the unborn child and the mother, and on condition that the parents have given their free and informed consent to the procedure.* It follows that all research, even when limited to the simple observation of the embryo, would become illicit were it to involve risk to the embryo's physical integrity or life by reason of the methods used or the effects induced.

As regards experimentation, and presupposing the general distinction between experimentation for purposes which are not directly therapeutic and experimentation which is clearly therapeutic for the subject himself, in the case in point one must also distinguish between experimentation carried out on embryos which are still alive and experimentation carried out on embryos which are dead. *If the embryos are living, whether viable or not, they must be respected just like any other human person; experimentation on embryos which is not directly therapeutic is illicit.*[29]

No objective, even though noble in itself such as a foreseeable advantage to science, to other human beings or to society, can in any way justify experimentation on living human embryos or fetuses, whether viable or not, either inside or outside the mother's womb. The informed consent ordinarily required for clinical experimentation on adults cannot be granted by the parents, who may not freely dispose of the physical integrity or life of the unborn child. Moreover, experimentation on embryos and fetuses always involves risk, and indeed in most cases it involves the certain expectation of harm to their physical integrity or even their death.

---

document.

1) By *research* is meant any inductive-deductive process which aims at promoting the systematic observation of a given phenomenon in the human field or at verifying a hypothesis arising from previous observations.

2) By *experimentation* is meant any research in which the human being (in the various stages of his existence: embryo, fetus, child or adult) represents the object through which or upon which one intends to verify the effect, at present unknown or not sufficiently known, of a given treatment (e.g., pharmacological, teratogenic, surgical, etc.).

To use human embryos or fetuses as the object or instrument of experimentation constitutes a crime against their dignity as human beings having a right to the same respect that is due to the child already born and to every human person.

The Charter of the Rights of the Family published by the Holy See affirms: "Respect for the dignity of the human being excludes all experimental manipulation or exploitation of the human embryo."[30] The practice of keeping alive human embryos *in vivo* or *in vitro* for experimental or commercial purposes is totally opposed to human dignity.

In the case of experimentation that is clearly therapeutic, namely, when it is a matter of experimental forms of therapy used for the benefit of the embryo itself in a final attempt to save its life and in the absence of other reliable forms of therapy, recourse to drugs or procedures not yet fully tested can be licit.[31]

The corpses of human embryos and fetuses, whether they have been deliberately aborted or not, must be respected just as the remains of other human beings. In particular, they cannot be subjected to mutilation or to autopsies if their death has not yet been verified and without the consent of the parents or of the mother. Furthermore, the moral requirements must be safeguarded that there be no complicity in deliberate abortion and that the risk of scandal be avoided. Also, in the case of dead fetuses, as for the corpses of adult persons, all commercial trafficking must be considered illicit and should be prohibited.

5. How is one to evaluate morally the use for research purposes of embryos obtained by fertilization "in vitro?"

Human embryos obtained *in vitro* are human beings and subjects with rights: Their dignity and right to life must be respected from the first moment of their existence. *It is immoral to produce human embryos destined to be exploited as disposable "biological material."*

In the usual practice of *in vitro* fertilization, not all of the embryos are transferred to the woman's body; some are destroyed. Just as the church condemns induced abortion, so she also forbids acts against the life of these human beings. *It is a duty to condemn the particular gravity of the voluntary destruction of human embryos obtained "in vitro" for the sole purpose of research, either by means of artificial insemination or by means of "twin fission."* By acting in this way the researcher usurps the place of God; and, even though he may be unaware of this, he sets himself up as the master of the destiny of others inasmuch as he arbitrarily chooses whom he will allow to live and whom he will send to death and kills defenseless human beings.

Methods of observation or experimentation which damage or impose grave and disproportionate risks upon embryos obtained *in vitro* are morally illicit for the same reasons. Every human being is to be respected for himself and cannot be reduced in worth to a pure and simple instrument for the advantage of others. *It is therefore not in conformity with the moral law deliberately to expose to death human embryos obtained "in vitro."* In consequence of the fact that they have been produced *in vitro,* those embryos which are not transferred into the body of the mother and are called "spare" are exposed to an absurd fate, with no possibility of their being offered safe means of survival which can be licitly pursued.

6. What judgment should be made on other procedures of manipulating embryos connected with the "techniques of human reproduction?"

Techniques of fertilization *in vitro* can open the way to other forms of biological and genetic manipulation of human embryos, such as attempts or plans for fertilization between human and animal gametes and the gestation of human embryos in the uterus of animals, or the hypothesis or project of constructing artificial uteruses for the human embryo. *These procedures are contrary to the human dignity proper to the embryo, and at the same time they are contrary to the right of every person to be conceived and to be born within marriage and from marriage.*[32] *Also, attempts or hypotheses for obtaining a human being without any connection with sexuality through "twin fission," cloning or parthenogenesis are to be considered contrary to the moral law, since they are in opposition to the dignity both of human procreation and of the conjugal union.*

The freezing of embryos, even when carried out in order to preserve the life of an embryo—cryopreservation—*constitutes an offense against the respect due to human beings* by exposing them to grave risks of death or harm to their physical integrity and depriving them, at least temporarily, of maternal shelter and gestation, thus placing them in a situation in which further offenses and manipulation are possible.

Certain attempts to influence chromosomic or genetic inheritance are not therapeutic, but are aimed at producing human beings selected according to sex or other predetermined qualities. These manipulations are contrary to the personal dignity of the human being and his or her integrity and identity. Therefore in no way can they be justified on the grounds of possible beneficial consequences for future humanity.[33] Every person must be respected for himself: In this consists the dignity and right of every human being from his or her beginning.

II
INTERVENTIONS UPON HUMAN PROCREATION

By *artificial procreation* or *artificial fertilization* are understood here the different technical procedures directed toward obtaining a human conception in a manner other than the sexual union of man and woman. This instruction deals with fertilization of an ovum in a test tube (*in vitro* fertilization) and artificial insemination through transfer into the woman's genital tracts of previously collected sperm.

A preliminary point for the moral evaluation of such technical procedures is constituted by the consideration of the circumstances and consequences which those procedures involve in relation to the respect due the human embryo. Development of the practice of *in vitro* fertilization has required innumerable fertilizations and destructions of human embryos. Even today, the usual practice presupposes a hyperovulation on the part of the woman: A number of ova are withdrawn, fertilized and then cultivated *in vitro* for some days. Usually not all are transferred into the genital tracts of the woman; some embryos, generally called "spare," are destroyed or frozen. On occasion, some of the implanted embryos are sacrificed for various eugenic, economic or psychological reasons. Such deliberate destruction of human beings or their utilization for different purposes to the detriment of their integrity and life is contrary to the doctrine on procured abortion already recalled.

The connection between *in vitro* fertilization and the voluntary destruction of human embryos occurs too often. This is significant: Through these procedures, with apparently contrary purposes, life and death are subjected to the decision of man, who thus sets himself up as the giver of life and death by decree. This dynamic of violence and domination may remain unnoticed by those very individuals who, in wishing to utilize this procedure, become subject to it themselves. The facts recorded and the cold logic which links them must be taken into consideration for a moral judgment on *in vitro* fertilization and embryo transfer: The abortion mentality which has made this procedure possible thus leads, whether one wants it or not, to man's domination over the life and death of his fellow human beings and can lead to a system of radical eugenics.

Nevertheless, such abuses do not exempt one from a further and thorough ethical study of the techniques of artificial procreation considered in themselves, abstracting as far as possible from the destruction of embryos produced *in vitro*.

The present instruction will therefore take into consideration in the first place the problems posed by heterologous artificial fertilization (II, 1–3),* and subsequently those linked with homologous artificial fertilization (II, 4–6).**

Before formulating an ethical judgment on each of these procedures, the principles and values which determine the moral evaluation of each of them will be considered.

A. Heterologous Artificial Fertilization

1. Why must human procreation take place in marriage?

Every human being is always to be accepted as a gift and blessing of God. However, from the moral point of view a truly responsible procreation vis-a-vis the unborn child must be the fruit of marriage.

For human procreation has specific characteristics by virtue

---

*By the term *heterologous artificial fertilization* or *procreation*, the instruction means techniques used to obtain a human conception artificially by the use of gametes coming from at least one donor other than the spouses who are joined in marriage. Such techniques can be of two types:

a) *Heterologous "in vitro" fertilization and embryo transfer*: the technique used to obtain a human conception through the meeting *in vitro* of gametes taken from at least one donor other than the two spouses joined in marriage.

b) *Heterologous artificial insemination*: the technique used to obtain a human conception through the transfer into the genital tracts of the woman of the sperm previously collected from a donor other than the husband.

**By *artificial homologous fertilization* or *procreation*, the instruction means the technique used to obtain a human conception using the gametes of the two spouses joined in marriage. Homologous artificial fertilization can be carried out by two different methods:

a) *Homologous "in vitro" fertilization and embryo transfer*: the technique used to obtain a human conception through the meeting *in vitro* of the gametes of the spouses joined in marriage.

b) *Homologous artificial insemination*: the technique used to obtain a human conception through the transfer into the genital tracts of a married woman of the sperm previously collected from her husband.

of the personal dignity of the parents and of the children: The procreation of a new person, whereby the man and the woman collaborate with the power of the Creator, must be the fruit and the sign of the mutual self-giving of the spouses, of their love and of their fidelity.[34] *The fidelity of the spouses in the unity of marriage involves reciprocal respect of their right to become a father and a mother only through each other.*

The child has the right to be conceived, carried in the womb, brought into the world and brought up within marriage: It is through the secure and recognized relationship to his own parents that the child can discover his own identity and achieve his own proper human development.

The parents find in their child a confirmation and completion of their reciprocal self-giving: The child is the living image of their love, the permanent sign of their conjugal union, the living and indissoluble concrete expression of their paternity and maternity.[35]

By reason of the vocation and social responsibilities of the person, the good of the children and of the parents contributes to the good of civil society; the vitality and stability of society require that children come into the world within a family and that the family be firmly based on marriage.

The tradition of the church and anthropological reflection recognize in marriage and in its indissoluble unity the only setting worthy of truly responsible procreation.

2. Does heterologous artificial fertilization conform to the dignity of the couple and to the truth of marriage?

Through *in vitro* fertilization and embryo transfer and heterologous artificial insemination, human conception is achieved through the fusion of gametes of at least one donor other than the spouses who are united in marriage. *Heterologous artificial fertilization is contrary to the unity of marriage, to the dignity of the spouses, to the vocation proper to parents, and to the child's right to be conceived and brought into the world in marriage and from marriage.³⁶*

Respect for the unity of marriage and for conjugal fidelity demands that the child be conceived in marriage; the bond existing between husband and wife accords the spouses, in an objective and inalienable manner, the exclusive right to become father and mother solely through each other.³⁷ Recourse to the gametes of a third person in order to have sperm or ovum available constitutes a violation of the reciprocal commitment of the spouses and a grave lack in regard to that essential property of marriage which is its unity.

Heterologous artificial fertilization violates the rights of the child; it deprives him of his filial relationship with his parental origins and can hinder the maturing of his personal identity. Furthermore, it offends the common vocation of the spouses who are called to fatherhood and motherhood: It objectively deprives conjugal fruitfulness of its unity and integrity; it brings about and manifests a rupture between genetic parenthood, gestational parenthood and responsibility for upbringing. Such damage to the personal relationships within the family has repercussions on civil society: What threatens the unity and stability of the family is a source of dissension, disorder and injustice in the whole of social life.

These reasons lead to a negative moral judgment concerning heterologous artificial fertilization: Consequently, fertilization of a married woman with the sperm of a donor different from her husband and fertilization with the husband's sperm of an ovum not coming from his wife are morally illicit. Furthermore, the artificial fertilization of a woman who is unmarried or a widow, whoever the donor may be, cannot be morally justified.

The desire to have a child and the love between spouses who long to obviate a sterility which cannot be overcome in any other way constitute understandable motivations; but subjectively good intentions do not render heterologous artificial fertilization conformable to the objective and inalienable properties of marriage or respectful of the rights of the child and of the spouses.

3. Is "surrogate"* motherhood morally licit?

No, for the same reasons which lead one to reject heterologous artificial fertilization: For it is contrary to the unity of marriage and to the dignity of the procreation of the human person.

Surrogate motherhood represents an objective failure to meet the obligations of maternal love, of conjugal fidelity and of responsible motherhood; it offends the dignity and the right of the child to be conceived, carried in the womb, brought into the world and brought up by his own parents; it sets up, to the detriment of families, a division between the physical, psychological and moral elements which constitute those families.

B. Homologous Artificial Fertilization

Since heterologous artificial fertilization has been declared unacceptable, the question arises of how to evaluate morally the process of homologous artificial fertilization: *in vitro* fertilization and embryo transfer and artificial insemination between husband and wife. First a question of principle must be clarified.

---

*By *surrogate mother* the instruction means:

a) The woman who carries in pregnancy an embryo implanted in her uterus and who is genetically a stranger to the embryo because it has been obtained through the union of the gametes of "donors." She carries the pregnancy with a pledge to surrender the baby once it is born to the party who commissioned or made the agreement for the pregnancy.

b) The woman who carries in pregnancy an embryo to whose procreation she has contributed the donation of her own ovum, fertilized through insemination with the sperm of a man other than her husband. She carries the pregnancy with a pledge to surrender the child once it is born to the party who commissioned or made the agreement for the pregnancy.

4. What connection is required from the moral point of view between procreation and the conjugal act?

a) The church's teaching on marriage and human procreation affirms the "inseparable connection, willed by God and unable to be broken by man on his own initiative, between the two meanings of the conjugal act: the unitive meaning and the procreative meaning. Indeed, by its intimate structure the conjugal act, while most closely uniting husband and wife, capacitates them for the generation of new lives according to laws inscribed in the very being of man and of woman."[38] This principle, which is based upon the nature of marriage and the intimate connection of the goods of marriage, has well-known consequences on the level of responsible fatherhood and motherhood. "By safeguarding both these essential aspects, the unitive and the procreative, the conjugal act preserves in its fullness the sense of true mutual love and its ordination toward man's exalted vocation to parenthood."[39]

The same doctrine concerning the link between the meanings of the conjugal act and between the goods of marriage throws light on the moral problem of homologous artificial fertilization, since "it is never permitted to separate these different aspects to such a degree as positively to exclude either the procreative intention or the conjugal relation."[40]

Contraception deliberately deprives the conjugal act of its openness to procreation and in this way brings about a voluntary dissociation of the ends of marriage. Homologous artificial fertilization, in seeking a procreation which is not the fruit of a specific act of conjugal union, objectively effects an analogous separation between the goods and the meanings of marriage.

Thus *fertilization is licitly sought when it is the result of a "conjugal act which is per se suitable for the generation of children, to which marriage is ordered by its nature and by which the spouses become one flesh."*[41] *But from the moral point of view procreation is deprived of its proper perfection when it is not desired as the fruit of the conjugal act, that is to say, of the specific act of the spouses' union.*

b) The moral value of the intimate link between the goods of marriage and between the meanings of the conjugal act is based upon the unity of the human being, a unity involving body and spiritual soul.[42] Spouses mutually express their personal love in the "language of the body," which clearly involves both "spousal meanings" and parental ones.[43] The conjugal act by which the couple mutually express their self-gift at the same time expresses openness to the gift of life. It is an act that is inseparably corporal and spiritual. It is in their bodies and through their bodies that the spouses consummate their marriage and are able to become father and mother. In order to respect the language of their bodies and their natural generosity, the conjugal union must take place with respect for its openness to procreation; and the procreation of a person must be the fruit and the result of married love. The origin of the human being thus follows from a procreation that is "linked to the union, not only biological but also spiritual, of the parents, made one by the bond of marriage."[44] Fertilization achieved outside the bodies of the couple remains by this very fact deprived of the meanings and the values which are expressed in the language of the body and in the union of human persons.

c) Only respect for the link between the meanings of the conjugal act and respect for the unity of the human being make possible procreation in conformity with the dignity of the person. In his unique and irrepeatable origin, the child must be respected and recognized as equal in personal dignity to those who give him life. The human person must be accepted in his parents' act of union and love; the generation of a child must therefore be the fruit of that mutual giving[45] which is realized in the conjugal act wherein the spouses cooperate as servants and not as masters in the work of the Creator, who is love.[46]

In reality, the origin of a human person is the result of an act of giving. The one conceived must be the fruit of his parents' love. He cannot be desired or conceived as the product of an intervention of medical or biological techniques; that would be equivalent to reducing him to an object of scientific technology. No one may subject the coming of a child into the world to conditions of technical efficiency which are to be evaluated according to standards of control and dominion.

The moral relevance of the link between the meanings of the conjugal act and between the goods of marriage, as well as the unity of the human being and the dignity of his origin, demand that the procreation of a human person be brought about as the fruit of the conjugal act specific to the love between spouses. The link between procreation and the conjugal act is thus shown to be of great importance on the anthropological and moral planes, and it throws light on the positions of the magisterium with regard to homologous artificial fertilization.

5. Is homologous "in vitro" fertilization morally licit?

The answer to this question is strictly dependent on the principles just mentioned. Certainly one cannot ignore the legitimate aspirations of sterile couples. For some, recourse to homologous *in vitro* fertilization and embryo transfer appears to be the only way of fulfilling their sincere desire for a child. The question is asked whether the totality of conjugal life in such situations is not sufficient to ensure the dignity proper to human procreation. It is acknowledged that *in vitro* fertilization and embryo transfer certainly cannot supply for the absence of sexual relations[47] and cannot be preferred to the specific acts of conjugal union, given the risks involved for the child and the difficulties of the procedure. But it is asked whether, when there is no other way of overcoming the sterility which is a source of suffering, homologous *in vitro* fertilization may not constitute an aid, if not a form of therapy, whereby its moral licitness could be admitted.

The desire for a child—or at the very least an openness to the transmission of life—is a necessary prerequisite from the moral point of view for responsible human procreation. But this good intention is not sufficient for making a positive moral evaluation of *in vitro* fertilization between spouses. The process of *in vitro* fertilization and embryo transfer must be judged in itself and cannot borrow its definitive moral quality from the totality of conjugal life of which it becomes part nor from the conjugal acts which may precede or follow it.[48]

It has already been recalled that in the circumstances in which it is regularly practiced *in vitro* fertilization and embryo transfer involves the destruction of human beings, which is something contrary to the doctrine on the illicitness of abortion previously mentioned.[49] But even in a situation in which every precaution were taken to avoid the death of human embryos, homologous *in vitro* fertilization and embryo transfer dissociates from the conjugal act the actions which are directed to human fertilization. For this reason the very nature of homologous *in vitro* fertilization and embryo transfer also must be taken into account even abstracting from the link with procured abortion.

Homologous *in vitro* fertilization and embryo transfer is brought about outside the bodies of the couple through actions of third parties whose competence and technical activity determine the success of the procedure. Such fertilization entrusts the life and identity of the embryo into the power of doctors and biologists and establishes the domination of technology over the origin and destiny of the human person. Such a relationship of domination is in itself contrary to the dignity and equality that must be common to parents and children.

Conception *in vitro* is the result of the technical action which presides over fertilization. *Such fertilization is neither in fact achieved nor positively willed as the expression and fruit of a specific act of the conjugal union. In homologous "in vitro" fertilization and embryo transfer, therefore, even if it is considered in the context of de facto existing sexual relations, the generation of the human person is objectively deprived of its proper perfection: namely, that of being the result and fruit of a conjugal act* in which the spouses can become "cooperators with God for giving life to a new person."[50]

These reasons enable us to understand why the act of conjugal love is considered in the teaching of the church as the only setting worthy of human procreation. For the same reasons the so-called "simple case," i.e., a homologous *in vitro* fertilization and embryo transfer procedure that is free of any compromise with the abortive practice of destroying embryos and with masturbation, remains a technique which is morally illicit because it deprives human procreation of the dignity which is proper and connatural to it.

Certainly, homologous *in vitro* fertilization and embryo transfer fertilization is not marked by all that ethical negativity found in extraconjugal procreation; the family and marriage continue to constitute the setting for the birth and upbringing of the children. Nevertheless, in conformity with the traditional doctrine relating to the goods of marriage and the dignity of the person, *the church remains opposed from the moral point of view to homologous "in vitro" fertilization. Such fertilization is in itself illicit and in opposition to the dignity of procreation and of the conjugal union, even when everything is done to avoid the death of the human embryo.*

Although the manner in which human conception is achieved with *in vitro* fertilization and embryo transfer cannot be approved, every child which comes into the world must in any case be accepted as a living gift of the divine Goodness and must be brought up with love.

6. How is homologous artificial insemination to be evaluated from the moral point of view?

Homologous artificial insemination within marriage cannot be admitted except for those cases in which the technical means is not a substitute for the conjugal act but serves to facilitate and to help so that the act attains its natural purpose.

The teaching of the magisterium on this point has already been stated.[51] This teaching is not just an expression of particular historical circumstances, but is based on the church's doctrine concerning the connection between the conjugal union and procreation and on a consideration of the personal nature of the conjugal act and of human procreation. "In its natural structure, the conjugal act is a personal action, a simultaneous and immediate cooperation on the part of the husband and wife, which by the very nature of the agents and the proper nature of the act is the expression of the mutual gift which, according to the words of Scripture, brings about union 'in one flesh' "[52] Thus moral conscience "does not necessarily proscribe the use of certain artificial means destined solely either to the facilitating of the natural act or to ensuring that the natural act normally performed achieves its proper end."[53] If the technical means facilitates the conjugal act or helps it to reach its natural objectives, it can be morally acceptable. If, on the other hand, the procedure were to replace the conjugal act, it is morally illicit.

Artificial insemination as a substitute for the conjugal act is prohibited by reason of the voluntarily achieved dissociation of the two meanings of the conjugal act. Masturbation, through which the sperm is normally obtained, is another sign of this dissociation: Even when it is done for the purpose of procreation the act remains deprived of its unitive meaning: "It lacks the sexual relationship called for by the moral order, namely the relationship which realizes 'the full sense of mutual self-giving and human procreation in the context of true love.' "[54]

7. What moral criterion can be proposed with regard to medical intervention in human procreation?

The medical act must be evaluated not only with reference to its technical dimension, but also and above all in relation to its goal, which is the good of persons and their bodily and psychological health. The moral criteria for medical intervention in procreation are deduced from the dignity of human persons, of their sexuality and of their origin.

Medicine which seeks to be ordered to the integral good of the person must respect the specifically human values of sexuality.[55] The doctor is at the service of persons and of human procreation. He does not have the authority to dispose of them or to decide their fate. A medical intervention respects the dignity of persons when it seeks to assist the conjugal act either in order to facilitate its performance or in order to enable it to achieve its objective once it has been normally performed.[56]

On the other hand, it sometimes happens that a medical procedure technologically replaces the conjugal act in order to obtain a procreation which is neither its result nor its fruit. In this case the medical act is not, as it should be, at the service of conjugal union, but rather appropriates to itself the procreative function and thus contradicts the dignity and the inalienable rights of the spouses and of the child to be born.

The humanization of medicine, which is insisted upon today by everyone, requires respect for the integral dignity of the human person first of all in the act and at the moment in which the spouses transmit life to a new person. It is only logical therefore to address an urgent appeal to Catholic doctors and scientists that they bear exemplary witness to the respect due to the human embryo and to the dignity of procreation. The medical and nursing staff of Catholic hospitals and clinics are in a special way urged to do justice to the moral obligations which they have assumed, frequently also, as part of their contract. Those who are in charge of Catholic hospitals and clinics and who are often religious will take special care to safeguard and promote a diligent observance of the moral norms recalled in the present instruction.

8. The suffering caused by infertility in marriage.

The suffering of spouses who cannot have children or who are afraid of bringing a handicapped child into the world is a suffering that everyone must understand and properly evaluate.

On the part of the spouses, the desire for a child is natural: It expresses the vocation to fatherhood and motherhood inscribed in conjugal love. This desire can be even stronger if the couple is affected by sterility which appears incurable. Nevertheless, marriage does not confer upon the spouses the right to have a child, but only the right to perform those natural acts which are per se ordered to procreation.[57]

A true and proper right to a child would be contrary to the child's dignity and nature. The child is not an object to which one has a right nor can he be considered as an object of ownership: Rather, a child is a gift, "the supreme gift"[58] and the most gratuitous gift of marriage, and is a living testimony of the mutual giving of his parents. For this reason, the child has the right as already mentioned, to be the fruit of the specific act of the conjugal love of his parents; and he also has the right to be respected as a person from the moment of his conception.

Nevertheless, whatever its cause or prognosis, sterility is certainly a difficult trial. The community of believers is called to shed light upon and support the suffering of those who are unable to fulfill their legitimate aspiration to motherhood and fatherhood. Spouses who find themselves in this sad situation are called to find in it an opportunity for sharing in a particular way in the Lord's cross, the source of spiritual fruitfulness. Sterile couples must not forget that "even when procreation is not possible, conjugal life does not for this reason lose its value. Physical sterility in fact can be for spouses the occasion for other important services to the life of the human person, for example, adoption, various forms of educational work and assistance to other families and to poor or handicapped children."[59]

Many researchers are engaged in the fight against sterility. While fully safeguarding the dignity of human procreation, some have achieved results which previously seemed unattainable. Scientists therefore are to be encouraged to continue their research with the aim of preventing the causes of sterility and of being able to remedy them so that sterile couples will be able to procreate in full respect for their own personal dignity and that of the child to be born.

III
MORAL AND CIVIL LAW

The Values and Moral Obligations That Civil Legislation Must Respect And Sanction in This Matter

The inviolable right to life of every innocent human individual and the rights of the family and of the institution of marriage constitute fundamental moral values because they concern the natural condition and integral vocation of the human person; at the same time they are constitutive elements of civil society and its order.

For this reason the new technological possibilities which have opened up in the field of biomedicine require the intervention of the political authorities and of the legislator, since an uncontrolled application of such techniques could lead to unforeseeable and damaging consequences for civil society. Recourse to the conscience of each individual and to the self-regulation of researchers cannot be sufficient for ensuring respect for personal rights and public order. If the legislator responsible for the common good were not watchful, he could be deprived of his prerogatives by researchers claiming to govern humanity in the name of the biological discoveries and the alleged "improvement" processes which they would draw from those discoveries. "Eugenism" and forms of discrimination between human beings could come to be legitimized: This would constitute an act of violence and a serious offense to the equality, dignity and fundamental rights of the human person.

The intervention of the public authority must be inspired by the rational principles which regulate the relationships between civil law and moral law. The task of the civil law is to ensure the common good of people through the recognition of and the defense of fundamental rights and through the promotion of peace and of public morality.[60] In no sphere of life can the civil law take the place of conscience or dictate norms concerning things which are outside its competence. It must sometimes tolerate, for the sake of public order, things which it cannot forbid without a greater evil resulting. However, the inalienable rights of the person must be recognized and respected by civil society and the political authority. These human rights depend neither on single individuals nor on parents; nor do they represent a concession made by society and the state: They pertain to human nature and are inherent in the person by virtue of the creative act from which the person took his or her origin.

Among such fundamental rights one should mention in this regard: a) every human being's right to life and physical integrity from the moment of conception until death; b) the rights of the family and of marriage as an institution and, in this area, the child's right to be conceived, brought into the world and brought up by his parents. To each of these two themes it is necessary here to give some further consideration.

In various states certain laws have authorized the direct suppression of innocents: The moment a positive law deprives a category of human beings of the protection which civil legislation must accord them, the state is denying the equality of all before the law. When the state does not place its power at the service of the rights of each citizen, and in particular of the more vulnerable, the very foundations of a state based on law are undermined. The political authority consequently cannot give approval to the calling of human beings into existence through procedures which would expose them to those very grave risks noted previously. The possible recognition by positive law and the political authorities of techniques of artificial transmission of life and the experimentation connected with it would widen the breach already opened by the legalization of abortion.

As a consequence of the respect and protection which must be ensured for the unborn child from the moment of his conception, the law must provide appropriate penal sanctions for every deliberate violation of the child's rights. The law cannot tolerate—indeed it must expressly forbid—that human beings, even at the embryonic stage, should be treated as objects of experimentation, be mutilated or destroyed with the excuse that they are superfluous or incapable of developing normally.

The political authority is bound to guarantee to the institution of the family, upon which society is based, the juridical protection to which it has a right. From the very fact that it is at the service of people, the political authority must also be at the service of the family. Civil law cannot grant approval to techniques of artificial procreation which, for the benefit of third parties (doctors, biologists, economic or governmental powers), take away what is a right inherent in the relationship between spouses; and therefore civil law cannot legalize the donation of gametes between persons who are not legitimately united in marriage.

Legislation must also prohibit, by virtue of the support which is due to the family, embryo banks, post-mortem insemination and "surrogate motherhood."

It is part of the duty of the public authority to ensure that the civil law is regulated according to the fundamental norms of the moral law in matters concerning human rights, human life and the institution of the family. Politicians must commit themselves, through their interventions upon public opinion, to securing in society the widest possible consensus on such essential points and to consolidating this consensus wherever it risks being weakened or is in danger of collapse.

In many countries the legalization of abortion and juridical tolerance of unmarried couples make it more difficult to secure respect for the fundamental rights recalled by this instruction. It is to be hoped that states will not become responsible for aggravating these socially damaging situations of injustice. It is rather to be hoped that nations and states will realize all the cultural, ideological and political implications connected with the techniques of artificial procreation and will find the wisdom and courage necessary for issuing laws which are more just and more respectful of human life and the institution of the family.

The civil legislation of many states confers an undue legitimation upon certain practices in the eyes of many today; it is seen to be incapable of guaranteeing that morality which is in conformity with the natural exigencies of the human person and with the "unwritten laws" etched by the Creator upon the human heart. All men of good will must commit themselves, particularly within their professional field and in the exercise of their civil rights, to ensuring the reform of morally unacceptable civil laws and the correction of illicit practices. In addition, "conscientious objection" vis-a-vis such laws must be supported and recognized. A movement of passive resistance to the legitimation of practices contrary to human life and dignity is beginning to make an ever sharper impression upon the moral conscience of many, especially among specialists in the biomedical sciences.

CONCLUSION

The spread of technologies of intervention in the processes of human procreation raises very serious moral problems in relation to the respect due to the human being from the moment of conception, to the dignity of the person, of his or her sexuality and of the transmission of life.

With this instruction the Congregation for the Doctrine of the Faith, in fulfilling its responsibility to promote and defend the church's teaching in so serious a matter, addresses a new and heartfelt invitation to all those who, by reason of their role and their commitment, can exercise a positive influence and ensure that in the family and in society due respect is accorded to life and love. It addresses this invitation to those responsible for the formation of consciences and of public opinion, to scientists and medical professionals, to jurists and politicians. It hopes that all will understand the incompatibility between recognition of the dignity of the human person and contempt for life and love, between faith in the living God and the claim to decide arbitrarily the origin and fate of a human being.

In particular, the Congregation for the Doctrine of the Faith addresses an invitation with confidence and encouragement to theologians, and above all to moralists, that they study more deeply and make ever more accessible to the faithful the contents of the teaching of the church's magisterium in the light of a valid anthropology in the matter of sexuality and marriage and in the context of the necessary interdisciplinary approach. Thus they will make it possible to understand ever more clearly the reasons for and the validity of this teaching. By defending man against the excesses of his own power, the church of God reminds him of the reasons for his true nobility; only in this way can the possibility of living and loving with that dignity and liberty which derive from respect for the truth be ensured for the men and women of tomorrow. The precise indications which are offered in the present instruction therefore are not meant to halt the effort of reflection, but rather to give it a renewed impulse in unrenounceable fidelity to the teaching of the church.

In the light of the truth about the gift of human life and

in the light of the moral principles which flow from that truth, everyone is invited to act in the area of responsibility proper to each and, like the Good Samaritan, to recognize as a neighbor even the littlest among the children of men (cf. Lk. 10:29–37). Here Christ's words find a new and particular echo: "What you do to one of the least of my brethren, you do unto me" (Mt. 25:40).

During an audience granted to the undersigned prefect after the plenary session of the Congregation for the Doctrine of the Faith, the supreme pontiff, John Paul II, approved this instruction and ordered it to be published.

Given at Rome, from the Congregation for the Doctrine of the Faith, Feb. 22, 1987, the feast of the chair of St. Peter, the apostle.

Cardinal Joseph Ratzinger
Prefect

Archbishop Alberto Bovone
Secretary

Notes

1. Pope John Paul II, Discourse to those taking part in the 81st Congress of the Italian Society of Internal Medicine and the 82nd Congress of the Italian Society of General Surgery, Oct. 27, 1980: AAS 72 (1980) 1126.

2. Pope Paul VI, Discourse to the General Assembly of the United Nations, Oct. 4, 1965: AAS 57 (1965) 878; encyclical *Populorum Progressio*, 13: AAS 59 (1967) 263.

3. Ibid., Homily During the Mass Closing the Holy Year, Dec. 25, 1975: AAS 68 (1976) 145; Pope John Paul II, encyclical *Dives in Misericordia*, 30: AAS 72 (1980) 1224.

4. Pope John Paul II, Discourse to those taking part in the 35th General Assembly of the World Medical Association, Oct. 29, 1983: AAS 76 (1984) 390.

5. Cf. Declaration *Dignitatis Humanae*, 2.

6. Pastoral constitution *Gaudium et Spes*, 22; Pope John Paul II, encyclical *Redemptor Hominis*, 8: AAS 71 (1979) 270–272.

7. Cf. *Gaudium et Spes*, 35.

8. Ibid., 15; cf. also *Populorum Progressio*, 20: *Redemptor Hominis*, 15: Pope John Paul II, apostolic exhortation *Familiaris Consortio*, 8: AAS 74 (1982) 89.

9. *Familiaris Consortio*, 11.

10. Cf. Pope Paul VI, encyclical *Humanae Vitae*, 10: AAS 60 (1986) 487–488.

11. Pope John Paul II, Discourse to the members of the 35th General Assembly of the World Medical Association, Oct. 29, 1983: AAS 76 (1984) 393.

12. Cf. *Familiaris Consortio*, 11, cf. also *Gaudium et Spes*, 50.

13. Congregation for the Doctrine of the Faith, Declaration on Procured Abortion, 9, AAS 66 (1974) 736–737.

14. Pope John Paul II, Discourse to those taking part in the 35th General Assembly of the World Medical Association, Oct. 29, 1983: AAS 76 (1984) 390.

15. Pope John XXIII, encyclical *Mater et Magistra*, III: AAS 53 (1961) 447.

16. *Gaudium et Spes*, 24.

17. Cf. Pope Pius XII, encyclical *Humani Generis:* AAS 42 (1950) 575; Pope Paul VI, *Professio Fidei:* AAS 60 (1968) 436.

18. *Mater et Magistra*, III; cf. Pope John Paul II, Discourse to priests participating in a Seminar on "Responsible Procreation," Sept. 17, 1983, *Insegnamenti di Giovanni Paolo II*, VI, 2 (1983) 562: "At the origin of each human person there is a creative act of God: No man comes into existence by chance; he is always the result of the creative love of God."

19. Cf. *Gaudium et Spes*, 24.

20. Cf. Pope Pius XII, Discourse to the St. Luke Medical-Biological Union, Nov. 12, 1944: *Discorsi e Radiomessaggi* VI (1944–1945) 191–192.

21. Cf. *Gaudium et Spes*, 50.

22. Cf. ibid., 51: "When it is a question of harmonizing married love with the responsible transmission of life, the moral character of one's behavior does not depend only on the good intention and the evaluation of the motives: The objective criteria must be used, criteria drawn from the nature of the human person and human acts, criteria which respect the total meaning of mutual self-giving and human procreation in the context of true love."

23. *Gaudium et Spes*, 51.

24. Holy See, Charter of the Rights of the Family, 4: L'Osservatore Romano, Nov. 25, 1983.

25. Congregation for the Doctrine of the Faith, Declaration on Procured Abortion, 12–13.

26. Cf. Pope Paul VI, Discourse to participants in the 23rd National Congress of Italian Catholic Jurists, Dec. 9, 1972: AAS 64 (1972) 777.

27. The obligation to avoid disproportionate risks involves an authentic respect for human beings and the uprightness of therapeutic intentions. It implies that the doctor "above all . . . must carefully evaluate the possible negative consequences which the necessary use of a particular exploratory technique may have upon the unborn child and avoid recourse to diagnostic procedures which do not offer sufficient guarantees of their honest purpose and substantial harmlessness. And if, as often happens in human choices, a degree of risk must be undertaken, he will take care to assure that it is justified by a truly urgent need for the diagnosis and by the importance of the results that can be achieved by it for the benefit of the unborn child himself" (Pope John Paul II, Discourse to participants in the Pro-Life Movement Congress, Dec. 3, 1982: *Insegnamenti di Giovanni Paolo II*, V, 3 (1982) 1512). This clarification concerning "proportionate risk" is also to be kept in mind in the following sections of the present instruction, whenever this term appears.

28. Pope John Paul II, Discourse to the participants in the 35th General Assembly of the World Medical Association, Oct. 29, 1983: AAS 76 (1984) 392.

29. Cf. Ibid., Address to a meeting of the Pontifical Academy of Sciences, Oct.

23, 1982: AAS 75 (1983) 37: "I condemn, in the most explicit and formal way, experimental manipulations of the human embryo, since the human being, from conception to death, cannot be exploited for any purpose whatsoever."

30. Charter of the Rights of the Family, 4b.

31. Cf. Pope John Paul II, Address to the participants in the Pro-Life Movement Congress, Dec. 3, 1982: *Insegnamenti di Giovanni Paolo II*, V, 3 (1982) 1511: "Any form of experimentation on the fetus that may damage its integrity or worsen its condition is unacceptable, except in the case of a final effort to save it from death." Congregation for the Doctrine of the Faith, Declaration on Euthanasia, 4: AAS 72 (1980) 550: "In the absence of other sufficient remedies, it is permitted, with the patient's consent, to have recourse to the means provided by the most advanced medical techniques, even if these means are still at the experimental stage and are not without a certain risk."

32. No one, before coming into existence, can claim a subjective right to begin to exist; nevertheless, it is legitimate to affirm the right of the child to have a fully human origin through conception in conformity with the personal nature of the human being. Life is a gift that must be bestowed in a manner worthy both of the subject receiving it and of the subjects transmitting it. This statement is to be borne in mind also for what will be explained concerning artificial human procreation.

33. Cf. Pope John Paul II, Discourse to those taking part in the 35th General Assembly of the World Medical Association, Oct. 29, 1983: AAS 76 (1984) 391.

34. Cf. *Gaudium et Spes*, 50.

35. Cf. *Familiaris Consortio*, 14.

36. Cf. Pope Pius XII, Discourse to those taking part in the Fourth International Congress of Catholic Doctors, Sept. 29, 1949: AAS 41 (1949) 559. According to the plan of the Creator, "a man leaves his father and his mother and cleaves to his wife, and they become one flesh" (Gn. 2:24). The unity of marriage, bound to the order of creation, is a truth accessible to natural reason. The church's tradition and magisterium frequently make reference to the Book of Genesis, both directly and through the passages of the New Testament that refer to it: Mt. 19:4–6; Mk. 10:5–8; Eph. 5:31. Cf. Athenagoras, *Legatio pro christianis*, 33: PG 6, 965–967; St. Chrysostom, *In Matthaeum homiliae*, LXII, 19, 1: PG 58 597; St. Leo the Great, *Epist. ad Rusticum*, 4: PL 54, 1204; Innocent III, Epist. *Gaudemus in Domino*: DS 778; Council of Lyons II, IV Session: DS 860; Council of Trent, XXIV Session: DS 1798, 1802; Pope Leo XIII, encyclical *Arcanum Divinae Sapientiae*: AAS 12 (1879–1880) 388–391; Pope Pius XI, encyclical *Casti Connubii*: AAS 22 (1930) 546–547; *Gaudium et Spes*, 48; *Familiaris Consortio*, 19; Code of Canon Law, Canon 1056.

37. Cf. Pope Pius XII, Discourse to those taking part in the Fourth International Congress of Catholic Doctors, Sept. 29, 1949: AAS 41 (1949) 560; Discourse to those taking part in the Congress of the Italian Catholic Union of Midwives, Oct. 29, 1951: AAS 43 (1951) 850; Code of Canon Law, Canon 1134.

38. *Humanae Vitae*, 12.

39. Ibid.

40. Pope Pius XII, Discourse to those taking part in the Second Naples World Congress on Fertility and Human Sterility, May 19, 1956: AAS 48 (1956) 470.

41. Code of Canon Law, Canon 1061. According to this canon, the conjugal act is that by which the marriage is consummated if the couple "have performed (it) between themselves in a human manner."

42. Cf. *Gaudium et Spes*, 14.

43. Cf. Pope John Paul II, General Audience Jan. 16, 1980: *Insegnamenti di Giovanni Paolo II*, III, 1 (1980) 148–152.

44. Ibid., Discourse to those taking part in the 35th General Assembly of the World Medical Association, Oct. 29, 1983: AAS 76 (1984) 393.

45. Cf. *Gaudium et Spes*, 51.

46. Ibid., 50.

47. Cf. Pope Pius XII, Discourse to those taking part in the Fourth International Congress of Catholic Doctors, Sept. 29, 1949: AAS 41 (1949) 560: "It would be erroneous . . . to think that the possibility of resorting to this means (artificial fertilization) might render valid a marriage between persons unable to contract it because of the *impedimentum impotentiae.*"

48. A similar question was dealt with by Pope Paul VI, *Humanae Vitae*, 14.

49. Cf. *supra:* I, 1ff.

50. *Familiaris Consortio*, 14: AAS 74 (1982) 96.

51. Cf. Response of the Holy Office, March 17, 1897: DS 3323; Pope Pius XII, Discourse to those taking part in the Fourth International Congress of Catholic Doctors, Sept. 29, 1949: AAS 41 (1949) 560; Discourse to the Italian Catholic Union of Midwives, Oct. 29, 1951: AAS 43 (1951) 850; Discourse to those taking part in the Second Naples World Congress on Fertility and Human Sterility, May 19, 1956: AAS, 48 (1956) 471–473; Discourse to those taking part in the Seventh International Congress of the International Society of Hematology, Sept. 12, 1958: AAS 50 (1958) 733; *Mater et Magistra*, III.

52. Pope Pius XII, Discourse to the Italian Catholic Union of Midwives, Oct. 29, 1951: AAS 43 (1951) 850.

53. Ibid., Discourse to those taking part in the Fourth International Congress of Catholic Doctors, Sept. 29, 1949: AAS 41 (1949) 560.

54. Congregation for the Doctrine of the Faith, Declaration on Certain Questions Concerning Sexual Ethics, 9: AAS 68 (1976) 86, which quotes *Gaudium et Spes*, 51. Cf. Decree of the Holy Office, Aug. 2, 1929: AAS 21 (1929) 490; Pope Pius XII, Discourse to those taking part in the 26th Congress of the Italian Society of Urology, Oct. 8, 1953: AAS 45 (1953) 678.

55. Cf. Pope John XXIII, *Mater et Magistra*, III.

56. Cf. Pope Pius XII, Discourse to those taking part in the Fourth International Congress of Catholic Doctors, Sept. 29, 1949: AAS 41 (1949), 560.

57. Cf. Ibid., Discourse to those taking part in the Second Naples World Congress on Fertility and Human Sterility, May 19, 1956: AAS 48 (1956) 471–473.

58. *Gaudium et Spes*, 50.

59. *Familiaris Consortio*, 14.

60. Cf. *Dignitatis Humanae*, 7.

Notes

Chapter 1 / A Review of Artificial Reproduction

1. Ann Westmore, "History," in *Clinical In Vitro Fertilization,* ed. Carl Wood and Alan Trounson (Berlin: Springer–Verlag, 1984), p. 2.

2. Ibid.

3. Ibid.

4. Don P. Wolf and Martin Quigley, "Historical Background and Essentials for a Program in *In Vitro* Fertilization and Embryo Transfer," in *Human In Vitro Fertilization and Embryo Transfer,* ed. Don P. Wolf and Martin Quigley (New York: Plenum Press, 1984), p. 3.

5. Ibid., p. 4.

6. Westmore, "History," p. 8.

7. Linda R. Mohr and others, "Deep Freezing and Transfer of Human Embryos," *Journal of In Vitro Fertilization and Embryo Transfer* 2 (1985) 1–10.

8. David Malloy, M.D., and others, "A Laparoscopic Approach to a Program of Gamete Intrafallopian Transfer," *Fertility and Sterility* 47 (February 1987) 289–94.

9. Gary D. Hodgen, "Hormonal Stimulation for Fertilization *in vivo,*" in Wolf and Quigley, p. 251. Confer also Thomas J. O'Donnell, S.J., "New and Morally Acceptable Means to Overcome Female Infertility," *The Medical-Moral Newsletter* 20 (October 1983) 1–2.

10. John Biggers, "*In Vitro* Fertilization and Embryo Transfer in Human Beings," *The New England Journal of Medicine* 304:340ff.

11. Ibid., p. 340.

12. Ibid., p. 341.

13. John D. Biggers, "Risks of *In Vitro* Fertilization and Embryo Transfer in Humans," in *In Vitro Fertilization and Embryo Transfer,* ed. R. F. Harrison and others (London: The Academic Press Inc., 1983), pp. 393–409.

14. Ibid., p. 407.

15. Ibid.

16. Ian L. Pike, "Biological Risks of *In Vitro* Fertilization and Embryo Transfer," in Wood and Trounson, p. 141.

17. John L. Yovich and others, "Developmental Assessment of Twenty *In Vitro* Fertilization (IVF) Infants at Their First Birthday," *Journal of In Vitro Fertilization and Embryo Transfer* 3 (1986) 253–57.

18. Ibid., p. 255.

19. Ibid.

20. R. G. Edwards, "Current Status of Human *In Vitro* Fertilization," in *Fertility and Sterility: Proceedings of the XIth World Congress on Fertility and Sterility* (Lancaster, England: MTP Press, 1984), p. 110.

21. Alan H. DeCherney, M.D., "*In Vitro* Fertilization and Embryo Transfer: A Brief Overview," *The Yale Journal of Biology and Medicine* 59 (1986) 411.

22. Edwards, "Current Status of Human *In Vitro* Fertilization," p. 110.

23. Pike, "Biological Risks," p. 144.

24. John Leeton and John Kerin, "Embryo Transfer," in Wood and Trounson, pp. 128–29.

25. Yovich, "Developmental Assessment," p. 254.

26. R. F. Harrison and others, "Stress in Infertile Couples," *Fertility and Sterility,* pp. 369–76.

Chapter 2 / Sexuality, Marriage, and Parenthood: The Catholic Tradition

1. See especially Phyllis Trible, *God and the Rhetoric of Sexuality* (Philadelphia: Fortress Press, 1978).

2. See Walter J. Burghardt, S.J., ed., *Woman: New Dimensions* (New York: Paulist Press, 1977), especially chapters by Elisabeth Schüssler Fiorenza, Elizabeth Carroll, and Raymond E. Brown. See also Elisabeth Schüssler Fiorenza, *In Memory of Her: A Feminist Theological Reconstruction of Christian Origins* (New York: Crossroad, 1983).

3. See Victor Paul Furnish, *The Moral Teaching of Paul: Selected Issues*, 2nd ed. (Nashville: Abingdon Press, 1985).

4. For a historically situated treatment of the context of New Testament references to sexuality and marriage, see Pheme Perkins, "Marriage in the New Testament and its World," in William P. Roberts, ed., *Commitment to Partnership: Explorations of the Theology of Marriage* (New York: Paulist Press, 1987), pp. 5–30.

5. See Joseph A. Fitzmeyer, *To Advance the Gospel: New Testament Studies* (New York: Crossroad, 1981), pp. 79–111; John R. Donahue, "Divorce: New Testament Perspectives," *The Month* 14/4 (1981) 113–20; Pheme Perkins, "Marriage in the New Testament and Its World," pp. 15–20.

6. Tertullian, *Treatises on Marriage and Remarriage: "To His Wife," "An Exhortation to Chastity," and "Monogamy,"* Ancient Christian Writers 13, trans. William P. Le Saint (Westminster, MD: Newman Press, 1956).

7. See Clement's "On Marriage," in *Alexandrian Christianity*, Library of Christian Classics 2, ed. John E. L. Oulton and Henry Chadwick (Philadelphia: Westminster, 1954), pp. 40–92.

8. Augustine, *Confessions,* trans. and ed. Albert Outler, Library of Christian Classics (Philadelphia: Westminster, 1955), VI, 15, 25; IX, 6, 14.

9. Augustine, *On Christian Doctrine,* trans. D. W. Robertson, Jr., Library of Liberal Arts (Indianapolis–New York: Bobbs–Merrill, 1958), p. 16.

10. Augustine, "On the Good of Marriage," 2, 13, in Roy J. Deferrari, ed., *St. Augustine, Treatises on Marriage and Other Subjects,* The Fathers of the Church (New York: Fathers of the Church, 1955). See also *Against the Two Letters of the Pelagians* and *On Marriage and Concupiscence,* cited in a valuable treatment of Augustine's views of sex, marriage, and sin by David F. Kelly, "Sexuality and Concupiscence in Augustine," *The Annual of the Society of Christian Ethics, 1983,* ed.

Larry L. Rasmussen (The Society of Christian Ethics, distributed by the Council on the Study of Religion, Wilfrid Laurier University, Waterloo, Ontario), pp. 81–116.

11. "On the Good of Marriage," 8.

12. Ibid., 6–7.

13. Ibid., 24.

14. Ibid., 1.

15. Thomas Aquinas, *Summa Theologica*, trans. by Fathers of the English Dominican Province (New York: Benziger, 1948), I-II, Q 94, a4.

16. Ibid., Suppl. 49; cf. 65.5.

17. Ibid., II-II, 26.11; *Summa Contra Gentiles*, trans. Vernon J. Bourke (Notre Dame: University of Notre Dame Press, 1975), 3/II, 123.

18. *ST* I.92.

19. *ST* I.91.1; *SCG* IV.88.

20. *ST* I.92.4.

21. *ST* I.92.1.

22. *ST* Suppl. 49, especially 3; 67.1; *St* II-II, 153.2; *SCG* 3/II.123, 126.

23. Michael G. Lawler, *Secular Marriage, Christian Sacrament* (Mystic, CT: Twenty-Third Publications, 1985), p. 37.

24. Ibid., p. 40. Lawler includes a more detailed discussion of the development of the sacramental and canonical status of marriage within Catholicism, with reference to the appropriate primary sources. A particular controversy had surrounded the moment of validity and indissolubility: consent or consummation.

25. Ibid., p. 46. Cf. canon 1013, 1.

26. Pius XI, *Casti connubii*, 273–74, in *Papal Teachings: Matrimony*, selected and arranged by the Benedictine Monks of Solesmes (Boston: St. Paul Editions, 1963). Pius XI here gives as his source St. Augustine, *De Gen. ad litt.*, 1, 9, c, 7, n. 12.

27. Ibid., 315.

28. *Gaudium et Spes*, 49, in *The Documents of Vatican II*, ed. Walter M. Abbott, S.J. (New York: America Press, 1966).

29. Ibid., sec. 50.

30. Robert Blair Kaiser states that "The council presidents made it clear to the council fathers they were to stay away from the birth

control question, because the pope was reserving the solution of that to himself and probably because the pope and some of his advisers were uncomfortable with the subject itself" (*The Politics of Sex and Religion: A Case History in the Development of Doctrine, 1962–1984* [Kansas City: Leaven Press, 1985], p. 63).

31. *Gaudium et Spes*, 51.

32. On the commission, its findings, and the development of the encyclical, see Robert G. Hoyt, *The Birth Control Debate* (Kansas City: National Catholic Reporter, 1968); and Robert Blair Kaiser, *The Politics of Sex and Religion*.

33. Paul VI, *Humanae vitae* (New York: Paulist Press, 1968), 11.

34. Ibid., 14.

35. Ibid., 7.

36. Ibid., 8.

37. Ibid., 9.

38. Ibid., 17.

39. The "Theology of the Body" series by John Paul II is published in three volumes by the Daughters of St. Paul (Boston). They are *Original Unity of Man and Woman: Catechesis on the Book of Genesis* (1981); *Blessed Are the Pure of Heart: Catechesis on the Sermon on the Mount and Writings of St. Paul* (1983); *Reflections on Humanae Vitae: Conjugal Morality and Spirituality.* (1984).

40. Quotations are from *Original Unity*, pp. 109–10, 119.

41. Ibid., p. 111.

42. *Reflections on Humanae vitae*, p. 33.

43. *Familiaris Consortio*, 32. The document is available from the United States Catholic Conference, 1312 Massachusetts Avenue, N.W., Washington, D.C.

44. Ibid., 22–23.

45. John T. Noonan, Jr., *Contraception: A History of Its Treatment by the Catholic Theologians and Canonists* (Cambridge: Harvard University Press, 1986), p. 533.

46. Ibid., p. 532.

47. See especially the comprehensive treatment by Ladislas Orsy, S.J., *Marriage in Canon Law: Texts and Comments, Reflections and Questions* (Wilmington, DE: Michael Glazier, 1986). Also valuable are Peter J. Huizing, S.J., "Canonical Implications of the Conception

of Marriage in the Conciliar Constitution *Gaudium et Spes,"* in William P. Roberts, ed., *Commitment to Partnership: Explorations of the Theology of Marriage* (New York: Paulist Press, 1987), pp. 102–36; Bernard Cooke, "Indissolubility: Guiding Ideal or Existential Reality?," in Roberts, pp. 64–75; Theodore Mackin, S.J., "How to Understand the Sacrament of Marriage," in Roberts, pp. 34–60; Ladislas Orsy, S.J., "Faith, Sacrament, Contract, and Christian Marriage: Disputed Questions," *Theological Studies* 43/2 (September 1982), 379–98.

48. 1983 Code, canon 1055, 1.
49. 1917 Code, canon 1081, 2.
50. Orsy, *Marriage in Canon Law,* p. 37.

Chapter 3 / An Overview of the Instruction

1. "Instruction on Respect for Human life in its Origin and on the Dignity of Procreation," Foreword. In the light of this claim, it is notable that there is no reference to any technical or scientific literature on artificial reproduction within the sixty footnotes. There are only three references to ecumenical councils (one each from Lyons and Trent and eleven from Vatican II; *Gaudium et Spes* is the only document from Vatican II cited and five of the eleven citations are to Paragraph 50). Two theologians are cited: Athenagoras and Chrysostom. No episcopal conferences are cited. All the other references are to encyclicals, papal allocutions and/or addresses, and documents from CDF.

2. James Burtchaell captures this shift nicely when he says: "The words are the words of Voltaire and Tom Paine but the thoughts are the thoughts of Jesus" ("The Natural Law Revisited," *National Catholic Reporter* 23 [8 May 1987] 12). The first part of the sentence is easily documentable. It may be a little more difficult to make an exact identification between the thoughts of CDF and the thoughts of Jesus.

3. "Instruction on Respect for Human Life," Introduction, 2.
4. Ibid.
5. Ibid., II, 7.
6. Ibid., Introduction, 1.

184 · *Religion and Artificial Reproduction*

7. Ibid., Introduction, 4.
8. Ibid., I, 1.
9. Ibid., I, 5.
10. Ibid., Introduction, 3.
11. Ibid., I, 2.
12. Ibid., note 27.
13. Ibid., I, 3.
14. Ibid., II, 1.
15. Ibid., II, 8.
16. Ibid.
17. Ibid., II, 1.
18. Ibid., II, 5.
19. Ibid., II, 4.
20. Ibid., II, 2.
21. Ibid., II, 4.
22. Ibid.
23. Ibid., I, 5.
24. Ibid.
25. Ibid., II, 2.
26. Ibid.
27. Ibid., II, 3.
28. Ibid., II, 4.
29. Ibid., II, 5.
30. Ibid., II, 4.
31. Ibid., II, 5.
32. Ibid.
33. Ibid.
34. Ibid.
35. Ibid., I, 6.
36. Ibid., II, 6.

Chapter 4 / A Comparative Analysis

1. For the most up to date picture of international guidelines on artificial reproduction, confer the special supplement "Biomedical Ethics: A Multinational View," *The Hastings Center Report* 17 (June 1987) 3ff. The first several articles provide an overview of the reg-

ulations in many countries and specific comments on individual countries.

2. The Department of Health, Education, and Welfare is now known as The Department of Health and Human Services (HHS). In this chapter I will continue to refer to these guidelines as the DHEW Guidelines since that was their original designation.

3. Ethics Advisory Board, U.S. Department of Health, Education, and Welfare, *Report and Conclusions: HEW Support of Research Involving Human In Vitro Fertilization and Embryo Transfer* (Washington, D.C.: U.S. Government Printing Office, 1979). This book is out of print. The Regulations are also available in the *Federal Register* 44 (18 June 1979) 35033-58. A more accessible source of the DHEW conclusions is Peter Singer and Deane Wells, *Making Babies: The New Science and Ethics of Conception* (New York: Scribner's, 1985). Since this book also contains the Australian and British guidelines, I refer to it for those citations as well.

4. Singer and Wells, *Making Babies,* p. 183.

5. Ibid., p. 184.

6. Ibid.

7. Ibid.

8. Ibid., p. 185.

9. Ibid.

10. Ibid.

11. Ibid., p. 187.

12. "Ethical Issues in Surrogate Motherhood" (The American College of Obstetricians and Gynecologists, 600 Maryland Ave., S.W., Suite 300 East, Washington, D.C. 20024).

13. Ibid.

14. The Ethics Committee of the American Fertility Society, "Ethical Considerations of the New Reproductive Technologies." *Fertility and Sterility* 46 (September 1987).

15. A critical question may have been begged at the very beginning of the report when the Committee says the procedures are to be offered ". . . only if they provide a reasonable chance of solving the *medical* problem" (ibid., p. v., emphasis added). If the *medical* problem is infertility, the reproductive technologies do not resolve that problem. They resolve only *childlessness.* If one is infertile before

IVF and ET, preembryo lavage or surrogacy, one is infertile afterwards. The unresolved question, in my judgement, is in what sense do the reproductive technologies fit into the traditional medical model?

16. Ibid., p. 1S. Emphasis in the original.
17. Ibid.
18. Ibid.
19. Ibid.
20. Ibid., p. 2S.
21. Ibid., p. 6S.
22. Ibid., p. 21S.
23. Ibid., p. 22S.
24. A preembryo is a "product of gametic union from fertilization to the appearance of the embryonic axis. The preembryonic stage is considered to last until 14 days after fertilization" (ibid., p. vii).
25. Ibid., pp. 29S–30S.
26. Ibid., p. 30S.
27. Ibid., pp. 24S–25S.
28. Ibid., p. 33S.
29. Ibid., p. 37S. There is a note here that this conclusion is too assertive and unnuanced. The suggestion is made that the conclusion would more appropriately read: "The Committee finds AID not clearly and certainly unethical" (ibid.).
30. Ibid., p. 39S.
31. Ibid.
32. Ibid., p. 44S.
33. Ibid., p. 46S.
34. Ibid., p. 48S.
35. Ibid., p. 50S.
36. Ibid., p. 52S.
37. Ibid., p. 53S.
38. Ibid., p. 55S.
39. Ibid., pp. 58S–9S.
40. Ibid., p. 61S.
41. Ibid.
42. Ibid., 62S.
43. Ibid., p. 67S.
44. Ibid., p. 67S.

45. Ibid., pp. 69S–72S.
46. Singer and Wells, *Making Babies,* pp. 198–99.
47. Ibid., pp. 200–201.
48. Mary Warnock, *A Question of Life: The Warnock Report* (London: Basil Blackwell, 1984), p. ix. Emphasis in the original. Confer also the foreward to the report, pp. 1–3.
49. Ibid., p. x.
50. Ibid., p. 63.
51. Ibid., pp. 64–66.
52. Ibid., pp. 17–28.
53. Ibid., pp. 29–40.
54. Ibid., p. 47.
55. Ibid.
56. Ibid., p. 55.
57. Ibid., p. 56.
58. Singer and Wells, *Making Babies,* p. 191.
59. Ibid.
60. Ibid., pp. 191–192.
61. Ibid., p. 192.
62. Ibid., p. 193.
63. Ibid., p. 196.
64. Ibid.
65. Ibid., p. 197.
66. Louis Waller, "New Law for Laboratory Life," *Law, Medicine and Health Care* 14 (September 1986) 120–22.
67. Ibid., p. 121.
68. Ibid., p. 122.
69. "Instruction on Respect for Human Life," Introduction, 2.
70. Ibid.
71. Ibid.
72. Ibid., pp. 699–700. For an interesting evaluation of technology, confer Burtchaell, "The Natural Law Revisited," *National Catholic Reporter* 23 (8 May 1987) 10–11.
73. There are informal reports that many in the gay and lesbian community are successfully using artificial insemination outside of the medical context and that some clinics will artificially inseminate lesbians. Alternative reproductive clinics may be a logical outgrowth of this practice.

Chapter 5 / The Instruction as Roman Catholic Teaching

1. All the phrases quoted in this and the following paragraph are taken from the Introduction to the "Instruction on Respect for Human Life."

2. Francis G. Morrisey, O.M.I., "The Canonical Significance of Papal and Curial Pronouncements," 1981, Canon Law Society, Catholic University, Washington, D.C., 20064.

3. See Charles E. Curran and Richard A. McCormick, S.J., eds., *Readings in Moral Theology No. 1: Moral Norms and Catholic Tradition* (New York: Paulist Press, 1979); Richard A. McCormick, S.J., and Paul Ramsey, eds., *Doing Evil to Achieve Good: Moral Choice in Conflict Situations* (Lanham, MD: University Press of America, 1985); and Donald McCarthy, ed., *Moral Theology Today: Certitudes and Doubts* (St. Louis: The Pope John Center, 1984). A source of continuing value is the annual bibliographical review by Richard McCormick, "Notes on Moral Theology," appearing in the March issues of *Theological Studies*.

4. Contrast Richard A. McCormick, *Health and Medicine in the Catholic Tradition: Tradition in Transition* (New York: Crossroad, 1984), pp. 90–101; with Ronald Lawler, O.F.M. Cap., Joseph Boyle, Jr., and William E. May, *Catholic Sexual Ethics: A Summary, Explanation & Defense* (Huntington, Ind.: Our Sunday Visitor, Inc., 1985), pp. 151–75.

5. Contrast a favorable view, Lisa Sowle Cahill, "Teleology, Utilitarianism, and Christian Ethics," *Theological Studies* 42/4 (1981) 601–29; with a critical one, John Finnis, *Fundamentals of Ethics* (Washington, D.C.: Georgetown University Press, 1983), pp. 80–152.

6. Cited above, p. 182, m. 45.

7. "Instruction on Respect for Human Life," II, 1.

8. Ibid., II, 2.

9. Ibid., II, 5.

10. Ibid., II, 8.

11. Ibid., II, 5.

12. As we have seen, this monolithic approach does not trace back to Aquinas (see above, p. 38).

13. Although it cannot be denied that Catholic women have

abortions, many unwanted pregnancies among Catholics are attributable to the teaching against contraception. Schizophrenically, Catholic women (especially young ones) may refuse to use contraception because it is a "sin," but resort to abortion instead in case of conception.

14. See pp. 75.

15. Leon R. Kass, " 'Making Babies' Revisited," in Thomas A. Shannon, ed., *Bioethics,* 3rd ed. (Mahwah, N.J.: Paulist Press, 1987), p. 453. Originally published in *The Public Interest* 54 (Winter 1979) 44–51, 59–60.

16. Ibid., pp. 409–10.

17. Ibid., pp. 410–11.

18. *The New York Times,* 11 March 1987, A14–17.

19. See James Barron, "World Reaction: Views of the Vatican Document Vary from Approval to Vowed Resistance," *The New York Times,* 12 March 1987, B 11; and Paul Lewis, "Catholic Hospitals in Europe Defy Vatican on In-Vitro Fertilization," *The New York Times,* 18 March 1987, A1, A12.

20. Robert Suro, "Wide Appeal Made; Transfer of Embryos and Artificial Fertilization Largely Opposed," *The New York Times,* 11 March 1987, A 1.

21. Ari L. Goldman, "Some U.S. Dissent: Parts of Document Stir Sharp Disagreement from Theologians," *The New York Times,* 11 March 1987.

22. Ibid., A1.

23. Philip M. Boffey, "Effects on Couples: Doctrine Follows Years of Debate on Procedures," *The New York Times,* 12 March 1987, B11.

24. Robert Lindsey, "Catholics Who Want Children Are Seen as Ignoring Edict," *The New York Times,* 12 March 1987, B11.

25. Richard A. McCormick, "Op Ed: The Vatican Document on Bioethics," *America* 156/12 (28 March 1987) 147–48.

26. Richard A. McCormick, "The Vatican Document on Bioethics: Some Unsolicited Suggestions," *America* 156/2 (17 January 1987) 24–28.

27. Editorial, "New Vatican Instruction on Human Life and Procreation," *America* 156/12 (28 March 1987) 245.

28. Joseph Cardinal Bernardin "Science and the Creation of Life,"

The University of Chicago, 29 April 1987, in *Origins* 17/2 (28 May 1987) 21, 23–26.

29. Daniel E. Pilarczyk, "Taking it on the Chin—For Life: Reflections on a Vatican Instruction," *America* 156/14 (11 April 1987) 295–96.

30. James T. Burtchaell, C.S.C., "The Natural Law Revisited: Even Well-Engineered Humans Won't Live Happily Ever After," *National Catholic Reporter,* 8 May 1987, pp. 11–14, 19–21.

31. Ibid., p. 10.

32. Ibid., p. 20.

33. Ibid., p. 20.

34. Ibid., p. 21.

35. Charles Krauthammer, "The Ethics of Human Manufacture," *The New Republic,* 4 May 1987, p. 17.

36. Ibid., pp. 17–18.

37. Ibid., p. 20.

38. Ibid., p. 21.

39. For official statements, see William J. Gibbons, S.J., ed., *Seven Great Encyclicals* (New York: Paulist Press, 1963); and Joseph Gremillion, ed., *The Gospel of Peace and Justice: Catholic Social Teaching Since Pope John* (Maryknoll, NY: Orbis Books, 1976). For an interpretation, see David Hollenbach, *Claims in Conflict: Retrieving and Renewing the Catholic Human Rights Tradition* (New York: Paulist Press, 1979).

Chapter 6 / Conclusions

1. Cardinal Joseph Bernardin, "Science and the Creation of Life," Address at the University of Chicago, 29 April 1987, in *Origins* 17/2 (28 May 1987) 21, 23–26.

Index

191